D0746194

The Clinical Measurement of Joint Motion

Edited by

Walter B. Greene, MD
Professor of Orthopaedic Surgery
The University of North Carolina School of Medicine
Chapel Hill, North Carolina

James D. Heckman, MD
Professor and Chairman and John J. Hinchey, MD, Chair
Department of Orthopaedics
Medical School
The University of Texas Health Science Center at San Antonio
San Antonio, Texas

American Academy of Orthopaedic Surgeons
6300 North River Road
Rosemont, Illinois 60018

The Clinical Measurement of Joint Motion

Executive Director
Thomas C. Nelson

Director, Division of Education
Mark W. Wieting

Director, Department of Publications
Marilyn L. Fox, PhD

Book Design
Pamela Hutton Erickson

Production Manager
Loraine Edwalds

Assistant Production Manager
Kathy M. Brouillette

Publications Secretary
Geraldine Dubberke

The material presented in *The Clinical Measurement of Joint Motion* has been made available by the American Academy of Orthopaedic Surgeons for educational purposes only. This material is not intended to present the only, or necessarily best, methods or procedures for the medical situations discussed, but rather is intended to represent an approach, view, statement, or opinion of the author(s) or producer(s), which may be helpful to others who face similar situations.

Some drugs and medical devices demonstrated in Academy courses or described in Academy print or electronic publications have FDA clearance for use for specific purposes or for use only in restricted research settings. The FDA has stated that it is the responsibility of the physician to determine the FDA status of each drug or device he or she wishes to use in clinical practice, and to use the products with appropriate patient consent and in compliance with applicable law.

Furthermore, any statements about commercial products are solely the opinion(s) of the author(s) and do not represent Academy endorsement or evaluation of these products. These statements may not be used in advertising or for any commercial purpose.

First Edition
Copyright © 1994 by the
American Academy of Orthopaedic Surgeons

Library of Congress Catalog Card Number 93-74321
ISBN 0-89203-090-9

TABLE OF CONTENTS

Preface

The publication upon which this book is based, *Joint Motion: Method of Measuring and Recording* (1965), was significant in that it established a standard technique for measuring and recording joint motion. The Board of Directors of the American Academy of Orthopaedic Surgeons subsequently recommended publication of an updated version of this information, and two groups played an important role in its early development. Initial work was performed by a committee from the Council of Musculoskeletal Specialty Societies, whose members included John S. Gould (chairman), Paul A. Lotke, James W. Simmons, Jr., and Melvin Post. Subsequently, the Committee on Publications of the American Academy of Orthopaedic Surgeons participated in the development of this book. Members of the Publications Committee at that time included James D. Heckman (chairman), Benjamin L. Allen, Oren H. Ellis, Herbert Kaufer, Ronald L. Linscheid, James F. Richards, Jr., Dempsey S. Springfield, and Alan H. Wilde.

As work on this book evolved, it became apparent that a different focus was required. Many scientific studies on normal joint motion, accuracy of measurement and new methods of measurement have been published since 1965. Inclusion of some of this material was appropriate. Therefore, *The Clinical Measurement of Joint Motion* not only updates but also refines appropriate techniques for measuring motion of the spine and extremities and also discusses, where appropriate, normal joint kinesiology, the range of normal joint motion, and change in joint motion with age.

Measuring joint motion is an important factor in making clinical decisions. The methods described in this book were selected for their accuracy and practicality. We think that these techniques are applicable for the physician and therapist working in a busy clinic and, if used in a consistent fashion, will provide an efficient and objective assessment of joint motion that has reasonable accuracy and reasonable reproducibility.

The editors would like to acknowledge the many orthopaedic surgeons who have provided assistance and critique in preparing this book, and in particular the help of Vert Mooney, Bernard F. Morrey, and Thomas B. Dameron, Jr. In addition, the editors acknowledge Mark W. Wieting, Director of the Academy's Division of Education, who initiated and continued to encourage development of this project; Marilyn L. Fox, PhD, Director, Department of Publications, who directed the publication of this book; Pamela Hutton Erickson, who created the design and layout; Loraine Edwalds and Kathy M. Brouillette, who managed the production process; and Geraldine Dubberke, who provided word processing. We would also like to thank Nancy Place, of the University of Texas Health Science Center at San Antonio, who produced the illustrations; and Wiley Smith, of the University of North Carolina, who prepared the multiple revisions of the text.

Physicians and therapists who are evaluating and treating patients with musculoskeletal problems understand the necessity of a standardized, reproducible, and efficient method of measuring joint motion. We, the editors, hope that this book will facilitate that process.

Walter B. Greene, MD
Professor of Orthopaedic Surgery
The University of North Carolina
School of Medicine
Chapel Hill, North Carolina

James D. Heckman, MD
Professor of Orthopaedic Surgery
The University of Texas
Health Science Center at San Antonio
San Antonio, Texas

Purpose and Principles of Measuring Joint Motion

Measuring and recording joint motion is important for several reasons. In a patient with an acute injury or illness, the degree of joint mobility is an important clue to the correct diagnosis. For example, a two-year-old child with septic arthritis of the hip has a very different range of joint motion from a child of similar age who presents with transient synovitis. In both conditions hip motion is reduced, but the child with the infected joint will have a very restricted arc of motion, whereas loss of motion in the child with transient synovitis will be only 10° to 30°.

In chronic conditions, measuring joint motion provides an index to the severity and progression of the disorder. Loss of joint motion parallels loss of function in patients with chronic arthritides such as rheumatoid arthritis and hemophilic arthropathy.[1-6] Acute exacerbations of the synovitis in these disorders will likewise be heralded by decreased motion of the affected joint.

Measuring joint motion also provides important information concerning the results of treatment. We know that a pediatric patient with a septic hip is responding to therapy when the hip motion improves. Following extremity or spinal trauma, the range of joint motion is an important parameter in determining the return of an athlete to competition or a factory worker to the assembly line. Likewise, the analysis of a surgical procedure often includes comparison measurements of joint motion as an important indicator of results.

Measuring joint motion is an objective assessment that can be simply done. Therefore, when governmental or insurance agencies request a disability rating, the parameters for rating disorders of the extremity and spine are based largely on impairment of joint motion.[7]

Principles

Although joint motion can be visually estimated, a goniometer (Fig. 1.1) enhances accuracy of measurement[8] and is preferred at the elbow, wrist, finger, knee, ankle, and hallux. These joints allow palpation of bony landmarks and reasonably consistent alignment of the goniometer. A goniometer may also be used for measuring hip and shoulder motion. The overlying soft tissue, however, does not allow the same degree of repeatability when aligning the goniometer in these areas.

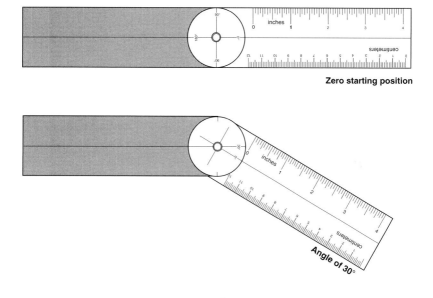

Zero starting position

Angle of 30°

Fig. 1.1A **GONIOMETER:**
Standard "pocket" goniometer with two arms that rotate around a central axis. Around this axis, one arm of the goniometer is marked in degrees.

Fig. 1.1B Moving the arms of the goniometer enables one to measure changes in joint motion.

The Clinical Measurement of Joint Motion

Measurement of joint motion must be performed and recorded in a consistent manner. Otherwise, communication among physicians and therapists will be inaccurate and ineffective. Obviously, defining the starting or zero position is most critical. The method used in this book is based on the Neutral Zero Position described by Cave and Roberts.[9] For most joints, the Zero Starting Position is the extended "anatomic position" of the extremity. To avoid confusion it is necessary to describe this position as 0° rather than 180°.

With the extremity in the Zero Starting Position, the central axis of the goniometer is positioned at the center of the joint. One arm of the goniometer is aligned with the proximal segment, while the other end of the goniometer is aligned with the bony axis of the distal segment (Fig. 1.2). The zero mark on the goniometer should be positioned over the distal segment. The upper or proximal end of the goniometer is held in place while the joint is moved through its arc of motion. The lower arm of the goniometer is then realigned with the axis of the extremity, and the degree of joint motion is read off the goniometer.

Joint motion is recorded as the maximum number of degrees a joint will move in a certain plane of motion. For example, the Zero Starting Position for the knee is with the leg extended

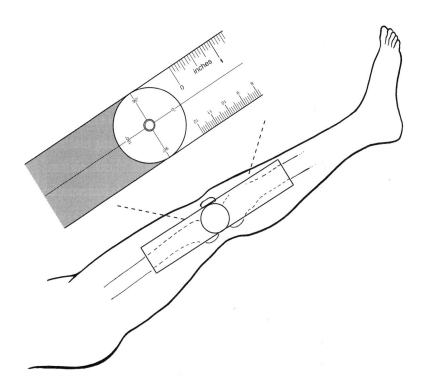

Fig. 1.2   **GONIOMETER** positioned to measure the extended extremity. One arm of the goniometer should be aligned with the axis of the proximal segment and the other arm should be aligned with the axis of the distal extremity. The zero-degree mark should be positioned on the distal segment. The proximal end of the goniometer is held in place while the joint is moved and the distal arm of the goniometer rotated. At completion of the movement, the degree of joint motion can be recorded from the goniometer.

straight. If a patient can bend the knee to 135°, the knee flexion would be described as 0° to 135° flexion or simply 135° flexion (Fig. 1.3).

Distinction is made between the terms "extension" and "hyperextension." Extension is used when the motion opposite to flexion is normal. Extension normally occurs at the wrist and shoulder joints. In addition, young children typically have some degree of extension of the elbow and knee.[10,11] However, if the motion is atypical, such as extension of the elbow or knee in an adult, or is asymmetrically increased at any age, it is referred to as hyperextension.

The terminology for describing limited motion of a joint is illustrated in Figure 1.4. The knee joint depicted in this drawing can be neither fully extended nor flexed. The restricted motion is recorded as follows: (1) the knee flexes from 30° to 90° (30°→ 90°), or (2) the knee has a 30° flexion contracture with further flexion to 90° (30° FC→ 90° or 30° FC W/FF 90°).

Joint motion can be measured as active or passive motion. To measure passive range of motion (PROM), the examiner moves the limb, but active range of motion (AROM) results from the patient's voluntary muscle contraction. With muscle weakness and/or arthritic changes, the patient will be unable to move the

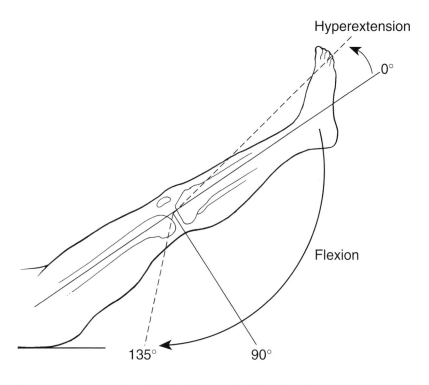

Fig. 1.3   **MEASUREMENT OF KNEE MOTION:**
Zero Starting Position: knee extended or straight with patient supine.
Flexion is measured in degrees from the Zero Starting Position.
Extension or Hyperextension is measured in degrees opposite to flexion at the Zero Starting Position.

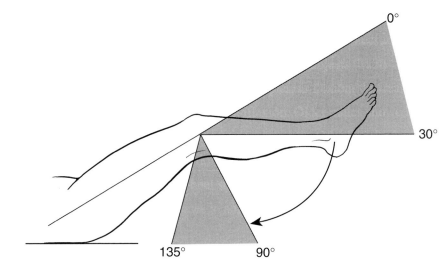

Fig. 1.4 **MEASUREMENT OF LIMITED MOTION OF THE KNEE:**

The terminology for recording limited motion of the knee is similar to that used at most, but not all, joints. (1) The knee flexes from 30° to 90° (30°→ 90°). (2) The knee has a flexion contracture of 30° with further flexion to 90° (30° FC → 90° or 30° FC W/FF 90°).

joint through its full arc of motion against gravity.
In that situation, active motion is different from the passive
range of motion. For example, if a knee joint can be passively
moved from 15° to 90° of flexion but lacks 30° of achieving
the Zero Starting Position on active extension, the arcs of active
and passive motion are different. The terminology for this
condition would be to list both active and passive arcs of
motion (30°→ 90° AROM, 15°→ 90° PROM).

Whenever possible, the motion of the affected extremity should
be compared with the opposite side. Many studies have confirmed that joint mobility of healthy subjects is equivalent on the
right and left extremity.[12-20]

Variability, as one would expect, is greater when a patient is
measured by different therapists or physicians. In a classic
study, Boone and associates[13] noted that intratester variability
accounted for approximately half the variability recorded when
different physical therapists made the measurements. With different examiners, Boone and associates[13] recommended that the
joint motion should differ by at least 5° before a true increase or
decrease in joint motion was recorded. Needless to say, it is
important to check the accuracy of the goniometer by validating
its measurements against known angles of 0°, 45°, and 90°.

The standard "pocket" goniometer is most widely used, but "scaled down" dorsal surface and lateral surface goniometers have been developed to measure finger motion (Fig. 1.5A). Likewise, a "universal" goniometer with longer arms has been developed for measuring large extremity joints (Fig. 1.5B). In an interesting study, Hamilton and Lachenbruch[15] did not find a significant difference between either dorsal surface, lateral surface, or the large "universal" goniometer when measuring finger joint motion.

Fluid-filled inclinometers can also measure joint motion (Fig. 1.6). Inclinometers are more expensive, relatively bulky, and vulnerable to being dropped, but they may be useful in measuring motion in certain regions such as the spine and hindfoot. Electronic goniometers have also been developed, but Clapper and Wolf [21] did not find that this device was more accurate than a standard goniometer.

Normal joint motion does vary among individuals, even those of the same race and gender. The range of normal motion also depends on the patient's age, gender, culture, and sometimes even on occupation. One might assume that females would have increased joint motion, secondary to greater ligamentous laxity. Indeed, this is sometimes noted,[17,22] but it is not observed at all joints or in all planes of motion.[16,17,23,24]

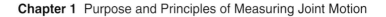

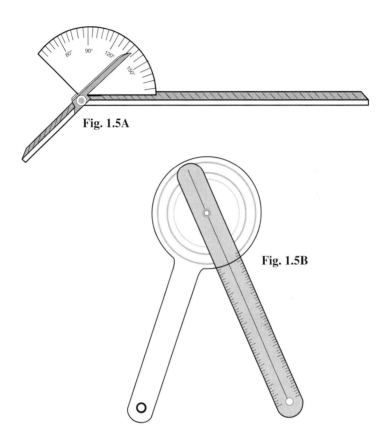

Fig. 1.5A

Fig. 1.5B

Fig. 1.5A   **SMALLER GONIOMETERS** may be useful in measuring finger motion. Diagram of a "scaled down" dorsal surface goniometer suitable for measuring finger joint motion.

Fig. 1.5B   **UNIVERSAL GONIOMETER** with long arms may be helpful in measuring motion at the hip, knee, elbow and shoulder, particularly in large individuals.

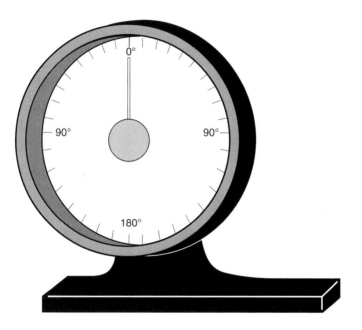

Fig. 1.6   **INCLINOMETER:** Fluid-filled with counter-weighted
needle maintains needle in constant vertical position. As the
joint moves, the dial is inclined or rotated and the degree of
motion can be measured.

Range of motion is slightly greater in children than in adults.[10,11,19] The total arc of motion gradually decreases as children get older. The increased joint motion seen in children is probably secondary to their greater ligamentous laxity, which also decreases as the child becomes older.[25] Decreased joint motion does occur as adults age, but the loss of motion is relatively small in most joints. Roach and Miles[24] analyzed hip and knee motion in healthy adults and found that the difference in motion between the 25-to-39-year-old group and the 60-to-74-year-old group ranged from 3° to 5° for each plane of motion. Restriction of movement may occur in older adults, and this is particularly common in females at the distal finger joints, but for many joints, it is safe to say that any substantial loss of mobility should be viewed as abnormal and not attributable to aging.

As a result of intrauterine packaging, neonates have striking differences in their range of joint motion. A typical newborn infant will have limitation of shoulder abduction, increased external rotation and decreased internal rotation at the hip, increased dorsiflexion and decreased plantar flexion at the ankle, and flexion contractures at the elbow, knee, and hip.[26,27] With the exception of the hip joint, a child will demonstrate normal range of passive motion by 3 months of age.[27] Increased external rotation and decreased internal rotation at the hip continue until a child is approximately 8 to 24 months old.[27-29]

Cultural differences may also affect the normal range of motion. Increased external rotation of the hips has been demonstrated in Saudi Arabian and Chinese populations, who spend extended periods of time in a squatting position.[12,30] Occupation may also influence the normal range of joint mobility. The most striking changes have been observed in professional ballet dancers, who show significant increase in knee extension and hip external rotation, flexion, and abduction with concomitant loss of hip internal rotation and adduction.[31] Changes noted in the ballet dancers are greater if their training and repetitive positioning began during early childhood.

Finally, motion of an injured or diseased joint is often painful. Every effort should be made by the examiner to be gentle. With an injured or diseased joint, it is best to record active motion first. This allows the examiner to gain some idea of the patient's discomfort. The examiner will then know how much support to provide the limb as the passive arc of motion is analyzed.

The Shoulder

The shoulder has greater mobility than any other joint in the body. The shallow socket of the glenohumeral joint is a key contributor to shoulder mobility. In addition, rotation of the scapula on the thorax positions the glenohumeral joints so that shoulder motion is significantly increased. Minor contributions to shoulder mobility include motion at the acromioclavicular and sternoclavicular joints.

Because the shoulder has an almost global range of motion, there are many positions and planes of motion that can be measured. Maximum shoulder motion, however, typically occurs as a composite movement rather than in a single plane of motion. For example, maximal elevation (flexion) of the shoulder can be achieved only as a composite movement that includes slight external rotation and abduction.[32]

Orthopaedic surgeons who specialize in treating shoulder problems typically limit assessment of shoulder motion to forward elevation (flexion), external rotation with the arm at the side, external rotation with the arm in 90° of abduction, and posterior reach (internal rotation with the arm at the side) as shown in Figs. 2.1–2.4. In addition to these four movements, the technique of measuring abduction, extension, and internal rotation with the arm abducted, (Figs. 2.1, 2.3 and 2.5) will be described. Abduction and extension may be helpful in describing a contracture or position of the shoulder that develops secondary to a neuromuscular or soft-tissue injury. Limitation of internal rotation with the arm abducted may be important with certain athletic injuries.

Measurements of shoulder motion are made with the patient in the standing position. If spine and pelvic motion cannot be controlled, external rotation and elevation should be assessed with the patient supine. The normal range of shoulder motion is listed in Table 2.1.

TABLE 2.1

RANGE OF SHOULDER MOTION
IN HEALTHY ADULT MALES*

Mean ± SD	
Elevation	167° ± 4.7°
Extension	62° ± 9.5°
External Rotation in Abduction	104° ± 8.5°
Internal Rotation in Abduction	69° ± 4.6°
Abduction	184° ± 7.0°

* Adapted from Boone and Azen.[14]

AROM was measured in 109 male subjects by methods developed in *Joint Motion: Method of Measuring and Recording*[33] with one possible exception. Elevation was described as flexion and perhaps did not permit enough external rotation and abduction to achieve the normal 180° elevation described by others.

Fig. 2.1   **ELEVATION (FLEXION):** The Zero Starting Position is with the arm at the side of the body. Elevation of the shoulder, sometimes called flexion or forward elevation, is the maximum upward motion of the arm. This motion includes flexion of the humerus and elevation of the scapula. Slight external rotation and abduction are also required to reach maximal elevation. These accessory movements are permitted, as it would be difficult to control or eliminate them when the shoulder is elevated. Furthermore, maximal elevation correlates better with functional impairment, eg, whether the patient is having difficulty getting a box off a high shelf. Normal shoulder elevation is 180°.[33]

EXTENSION: Extension of the shoulder, sometimes called posterior elevation, is motion in the opposite direction from forward elevation. Internal rotation is required for maximum extension.[32]

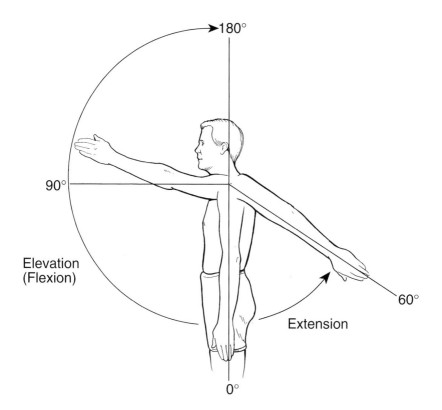

Fig. 2.2   **EXTERNAL ROTATION WITH THE ARM AT THE
SIDE (NEUTRAL POSITION):** The Zero Starting Position
is with the arm held comfortably against the thorax, the
elbow flexed at 90°, and the forearm parallel to the sagittal
plane of the body. The degree of external rotation is the maximum outward rotation of the arm from the sagittal plane. The
abdomen prevents accurate measurement of internal rotation
in this position. External rotation in neutral is often severely
restricted in patients with degenerative arthritis.

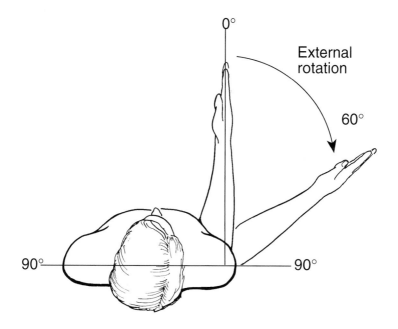

0°

External
rotation

60°

90°

90°

Fig. 2.3   **EXTERNAL/INTERNAL ROTATION WITH THE ARM IN 90° OF ABDUCTION:** The Zero Starting Position is with the arm abducted 90° and aligned with the plane of the scapula. The elbow is flexed 90°, and the forearm is parallel to the floor. External rotation in abduction is the number of degrees the forearm moves away from the floor. Limitation of external rotation in this position is seen in some athletes who emphasize strengthening exercises without including an appropriate stretching program and in patients who have undergone reconstructive operations of the shoulder via an anterior approach.

Internal rotation is the motion opposite external rotation; ie, the number of degrees the forearm moves toward the floor. If the arm is positioned posterior to the plane of the scapula, internal rotation will be restricted by mechanisms that are undefined but probably related to tightening of the glenohumeral capsular structures. Limitation of internal rotation in this position commonly occurs with problems of shoulder instability.

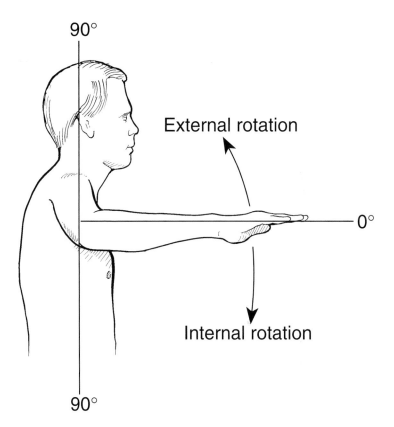

90°

External rotation

0°

Internal rotation

90°

Fig. 2.4   **POSTERIOR REACH (INTERNAL ROTATION):**
Posterior reach basically assesses internal rotation of the shoulder with the arm at the side. The maneuver, however, is a complex motion that is also dependent on shoulder extension as well as elbow, wrist, and thumb motion. Posterior reach is defined as the highest midline segment of the back that is reached by the hitch-hiking thumb. In healthy young adults, Kronberg and associates[34] observed posterior reach to the T4 level in females and to the T5 level in males. The editor's impression is that posterior reach in most adults usually ranges from the T6 to T10 spinous process. Patients with severe adhesive capsulitis or degenerative arthritis may have severe restriction of internal rotation. Posterior reach in these individuals may be described as "to the sacrum, gluteal region, greater trochanter, or lesser trochanter."

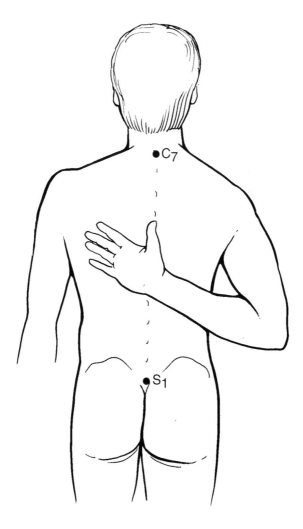

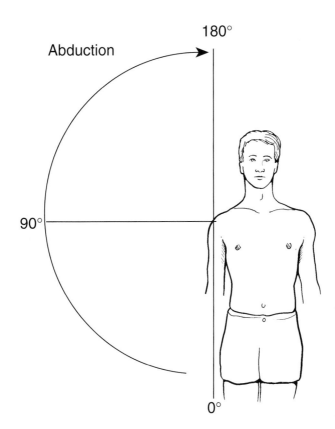

Fig. 2.5   **NEUTRAL ABDUCTION:** This is the upward motion of the arm in the coronal plane from the Zero Starting Position.

The Elbow

The elbow has three sites of movement: the ulnohumeral, the radiohumeral, and the radioulnar articulations. Description of elbow motion, however, is typically limited to the flexion-extension plane[33] for the following reasons: (1) forearm rotation involves motion at both the distal and proximal radioulnar joints and is, therefore, classified separately; (2) the radiohumeral and ulnohumeral joints are coupled so that as the elbow flexes and extends, similar motion is occurring at both articulations; and (3) movement in the other planes is minimal and inconsequential. Therefore, from a practical standpoint, the elbow can be functionally described as a uniaxial articulation centered at the ulnohumeral joint.[35]

The **Zero Starting Position** for measuring elbow motion is with the extremity straight (Fig. 3.1). Natural motion is flexion. The opposite motion beyond the Zero Starting Position is extension. Young children commonly extend the elbow by 10° to 15°, [10,11] but adults show minimal if any elbow extension (Fig. 3.2).

The normal range of elbow motion is listed in Table 3.1. Mild flexion contractures are of little functional consequence, as most activities of daily living are accomplished in an arc of elbow flexion from 30° to 130°.[37]

TABLE 3.1

NORMAL RANGE OF ELBOW MOTION

	Boone and Azen[14]*	Petherick and associates[36]**
Flexion	141° ± 4.9°	146° ± 6.3°
Extension	0.3° ± 2.0°	—

*   Subjects were adult males 20 to 54 years old.

**   Subjects were adults, male and female,

with an average age of 24 ± 4 years.

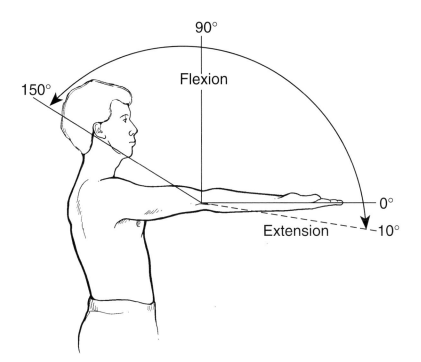

Fig. 3.1   **FLEXION AND EXTENSION:** The goniometer is centered at the anterior margin of the distal humerus to approximate the axis of elbow flexion-extension.[33] The arms of the
goniometer are aligned parallel to the axis of the humerus
and the forearm. Flexion: 0° to 150°. Extension: 0° to 10°.
Elbow extension is not present in all individuals.

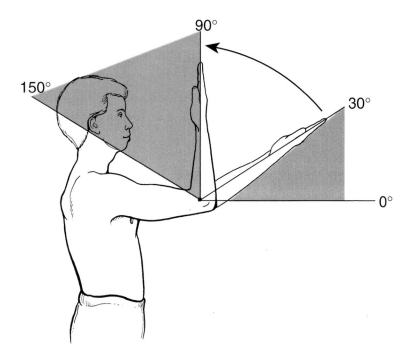

Fig. 3.2   **MEASUREMENT OF LIMITED ELBOW MOTION:**
The unshaded area indicates the range of limited motion.
Limited motion may be expressed in the following ways:
(1) the elbow flexes from 30° to 90° (30°→90°);
(2) the elbow has a flexion contracture of 30° with further
flexion to 90° (30° FC→90°).

Forearm Rotation

Forearm rotation is a composite motion occurring at the proximal and distal radioulnar joints, as well as the radiohumeral joint.[35] The plane of forearm rotation is pronation-supination. Pronation literally means "the state of being prone" or, as it relates to the forearm, "the palm being turned backward" (posteriorly). Likewise, supination literally means the "state of being supine," eg, the palm being turned forward (anteriorly).

Normal range of pronation and supination is listed in Table 4.1. Many activities of daily living are accomplished in the arc of motion between 50° pronation and 50° supination,[37] ie, the functional arc of forearm rotation. In addition, a very restricted arc of forearm rotation may be of limited consequence if shoulder mobility is normal and if the forearm is ankylosed in a neutral position.

To measure forearm rotation, the arm is stabilized against the chest wall, and the elbow is flexed to 90° (Figs. 4.1 and 4.2). The **Zero Starting Position** is with the extended thumb aligned with the humerus. To estimate pronation and supination, the examiner should palpate the radial and ulnar styloid as the forearm is rotated. Grasping a pencil or similar object facilitates visual estimation of forearm rotation. If a goniometer is used, one arm of the goniometer is aligned with the radially abducted thumb, while the other arm remains in a vertical position. An inclinometer may also be used to measure forearm rotation.

TABLE 4.1

NORMAL RANGE OF FOREARM ROTATION IN HEALTHY ADULT MALES

	Boone and Azen[14]*	Wagner[38]**
Pronation	75° ± 5.3°	71° ± 9.9°
Supination	81° ± 4.0°	88° ± 9.0°

*   Standard clinical measurement of AROM.

**   AROM measured in specially constructed apparatus.

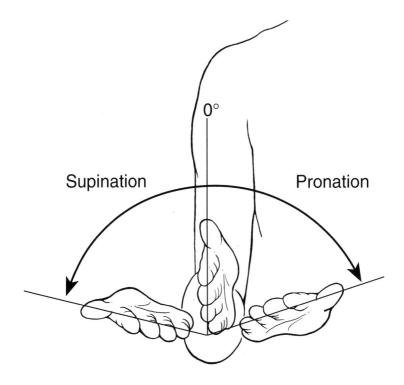

Fig. 4.1   **FOREARM ROTATION**

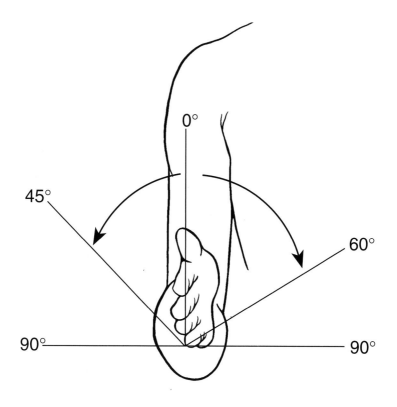

Fig. 4.2   **LIMITED MOTION**
Supination = 45° (0° → 45°)
Pronation = 60° (0° → 60°)
Total joint motion = 105°

C
H
A
P
T
E
R 5

The Wrist

Wrist motion is in the plane of flexion-extension (Fig. 5.1) and radioulnar deviation (Fig. 5.2). Flexion at the wrist is sometimes described as volar or palmar flexion, while extension is sometimes listed as dorsiflexion. Some degree of rotatory circumduction also occurs at the wrist, but this cannot be accurately measured in the clinical setting.

Wrist motion takes place at the radiocarpal and midcarpal joints. In a radiographic study by Sarrafian and associates,[39] motion at the radiocarpal joints accounted for 67% of wrist extension, while motion at the midcarpal joints made the greatest contribution to wrist flexion (60%). This pattern, however, showed some individual variation, with 27% of the subjects having a greater degree of flexion at the midcarpal joints, and 14% demonstrating a greater degree of extension at the radiocarpal joints.

In radial and ulnar deviation, the carpal rows rotate as linked segments. The buttress of the radial styloid limits radial deviation so that its arc of motion is significantly less than that of ulnar deviation (Table 5.1). Movement of the wrist into ulnar deviation is particularly important when performing activities of daily living.[40]

The instant center of motion for both flexion/extension and radial/ulnar deviation is located within the proximal pole of the capitate.[41] Therefore, when measuring wrist motion it is appropriate to align the axis of the goniometer with the proximal portion of the capitate.

TABLE 5.1

NORMAL RANGE OF WRIST MOTION IN HEALTHY ADULTS

	Boone and Azen[14]*	Ryu and associates[40]**
Flexion	75° ± 6.6°	79°
Extension	74° ± 6.6°	59°
Radial Deviation	21° ± 4.0°	21°
Ulnar Deviation	35° ± 3.8°	38°

*   Male subjects only.

**   Male and female subjects.

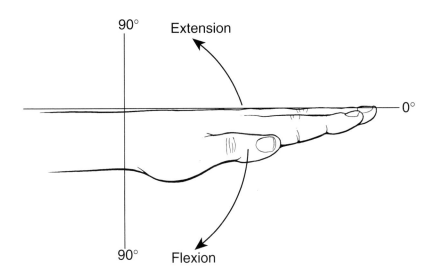

Fig. 5.1   **FLEXION AND EXTENSION:** With the forearm in
pronation, the **Zero Starting Position** is with the ulnar
border of the third metacarpal aligned with the axis of the
distal forearm. This position enhances positioning the axis
of the goniometer over the proximal capitate, ie, the center
of rotation for wrist movement. Measurements can be made
by placing the goniometer on the dorsum of the wrist or
by positioning it on the radial axis of the joint. If the
goniometer is aligned on the ulnar side, mobility of the
fifth metacarpal may falsely elevate the measurement of
wrist flexion-extension.

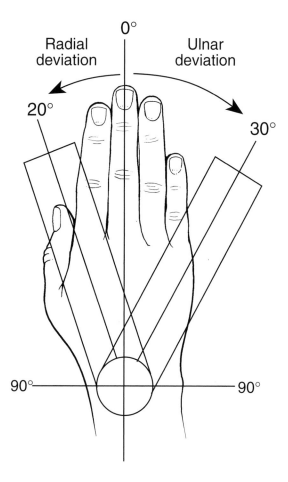

Fig. 5.2   **RADIAL AND ULNAR DEVIATION:** Zero Starting Position is the same as for measuring flexion and extension. Radial deviation equals 0° to 20°, ulnar deviation equals 0° to 30°.

The Hand

It is important to use correct nomenclature when measuring
and recording motion of the joints of the hand. In order to avoid
mistaken identity, the fingers and thumb are referred to by
name rather than by number. The metacarpals, however, are
referred to by number, with the first metacarpal being part of
the thumb, the second metacarpal articulating with the index
finger, and so forth (Fig. 6.1).

Each finger has four joints (Fig. 6.2): the distal interphalangeal
joint, abbreviated as DIP joint; the proximal interphalangeal
joint, abbreviated as PIP joint; the metacarpophalangeal joint,
abbreviated as the MP joint. Motion at the carpometacarpal
joints is not measured, being virtually nonexistent at the index
and long carpometacarpal joints and difficult to measure at the
more mobile fifth ray.

The thumb has only three joints (Fig. 6.3): the interphalangeal
joint, abbreviated as the IP joint of the thumb; the metacarpophalangeal joint, abbreviated as the MP joint of the thumb;
and the carpometacarpal joint, abbreviated as the CMC joint of
the thumb. Another name for the CMC joint of the thumb is the
metacarpotrapezial joint.

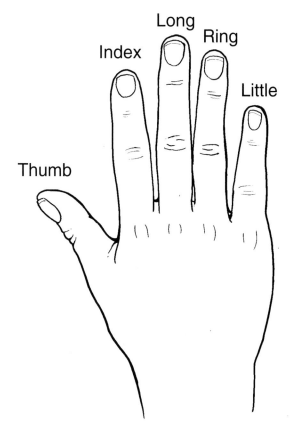

Fig. 6.1 NOMENCLATURE

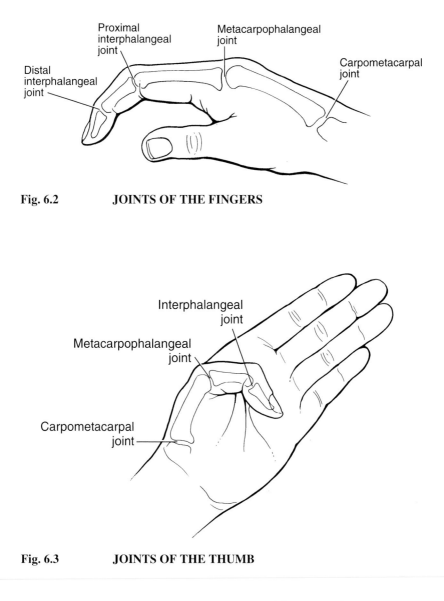

Fig. 6.2   **JOINTS OF THE FINGERS**

Fig. 6.3   **JOINTS OF THE THUMB**

The Fingers

Finger joint motion is primarily in the flexion-extension plane. Abduction and adduction are limited and occur only at the MP joints.

Flexion accounts for most of the motion of the finger joints (Figs. 7.1A–7.1C). Osteoarthritis often affects the DIP and PIP joints in older females and, therefore, older adult males often demonstrate a greater range of finger joint motion (Fig. 7.2). By comparison to young adult males, young adult females have a greater arc of finger joint motion primarily due to a greater range of extension at the MP joint.[17] In young adults, flexion of the digits is not affected by gender.[17]

Flexion of the MP joint increases in an approximately linear fashion as one progresses from the index to the little finger. At the PIP joint, flexion is equivalent for all digits, but at the DIP joint, active flexion of the ring and little fingers is less than the index and long fingers.[17]

Extension is greatest at the MP joints (Fig. 7.3), and at this joint is approximately equal for all digits.[17] Active extension is also equivalent for all digits at the PIP and DIP joints.

The position of adjacent joints is critical when measuring finger motion (Figs. 7.4–7.5). The wrist should be maintained in a neutral position. If the wrist is flexed, the extensor digitorum longus will be effectively tenodesed, thereby limiting flexion at the MP joints.[17] Likewise, if the PIP joint is maintained in extension, flexion at the DIP joint will be limited by 7° to 10°.

TABLE 7.1

ACTIVE RANGE OF FINGER MOTION
IN YOUNG ADULTS[a]

		Index	Long	Ring	Little
MP	Extension[b]	22°	18°	23°	19°
	Flexion[c]	86°	91°	99°	105°
PIP	Extension[b]	7°	7°	6°	9°
	Flexion[c]	102°	105°	108°	106°
DIP	Extension[b]	8°	8°	8°	8°
	Flexion[c]	72°	71°	63°	65°
TAM[d]	Males	284°	288°	294°	297°
TAM[d]	Females	305°	311°	318°	323°

[a] Adapted from Mallon and associates[17]

Subjects were 120 previously healthy adults between 18 and 35 years of age. The study had equal numbers of males and females and equal numbers who were right or left handed.

[b] Extension measured with fingers fully extended.

[c] Flexion measured after subjects had made a fist.

[d] Total active motion. Total arc of motion was greater in females by 21° to 26°. Greater extension at the MP joint made the greatest contribution to this difference in motion.

The Clinical Measurement of Joint Motion

Figs. 7.1A-7.1C   **FLEXION OF FINGER JOINTS,**
ZERO STARTING POSITION:
The wrist is maintained in the neutral position.

1A   **FLEXION AT THE DIP JOINT:** When measuring flexion at the DIP joint, the PIP joint should be flexed.

1B   **FLEXION AT THE PIP JOINT:** When performing this measurement, the MP joints can be positioned in either flexion or extension.

1C   **FLEXION AT THE MP JOINT.**

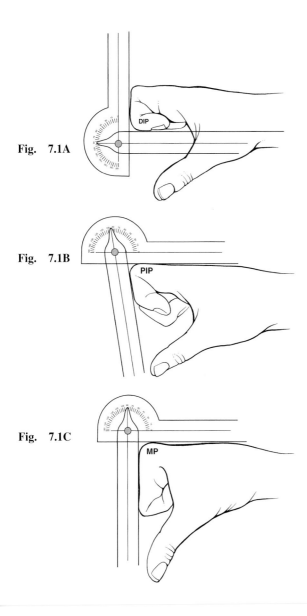

Fig. 7.1A

Fig. 7.1B

Fig. 7.1C

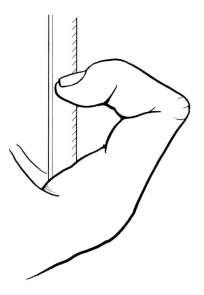

Fig. 7.2   **COMPOSITE MOTION OF FLEXION:** The distance
that the finger lacks in touching the distal palmar crease is a
simple maneuver and provides an informative measurement
of impaired finger flexion.

Chapter 7 The Fingers

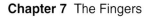

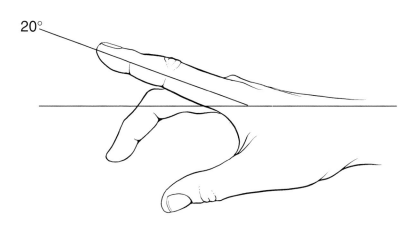

Fig. 7.3

EXTENSION: Extension is greatest at the MP joint and limited to an arc of 5° to 10° or less at the PIP and DIP joints.

It is useful to record the total active motion (TAM) and total passive motion (TPM). Total motion is the sum of flexion and extension occurring at the MP, PIP, and DIP joints.

For example:

Joint	Flexion	Extension
MCP	90°	-20°
PIP	100°	0°
DIP	35°	0°
SUM	225°	-20°
TAM	225° - 20° = 205°	

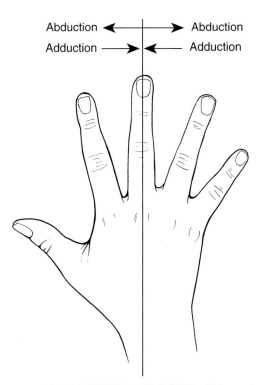

Abduction ◄——————►	Abduction
Adduction ——————►◄——	Adduction

Fig. 7.4   **ABDUCTION/ADDUCTION:** This motion is in the plane of the palm and is centered on the long finger. Abduction is movement of the fingers away from the long finger, while adduction is movement of the other fingers toward the finger.

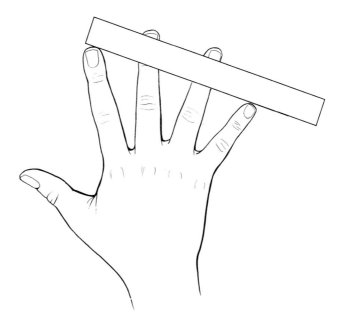

Fig. 7.5   **RANGE OF MOTION:** It may be described as the dis-
                     tance the fingers can be spread as measured from the tip
                     of the index finger to the tip of the little finger. Movement
                     between individual fingers may also be measured from tip
                     to tip of the indicated fingers.

The Thumb

Motions of the thumb are complex and reflect its overall importance to the function of the hand. This importance is also emphasized by the fact that a thumb amputation is rated as 40% impairment of the hand and 22% disability of the whole person.[7,42] The principal thumb motions are abduction, adduction, opposition, flexion, and extension.

Abduction and Adduction

Abduction of the thumb largely reflects motion at the carpometacarpal joint. It can be measured by the angle of the thumb and index metacarpal in both the palmar (Fig. 8.1) and radial planes (Fig. 8.2). Adduction of the thumb is the motion opposite radial abduction. This particular movement is usually not measured but is incorporated in the assessment of thumb opposition.

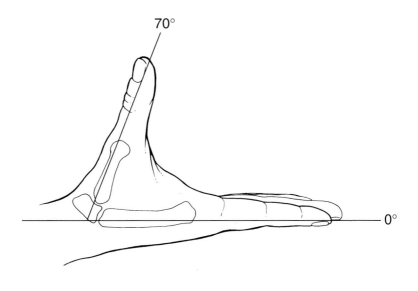

Fig. 8.1   **PALMAR ABDUCTION: ZERO STARTING POSITION.**
Palmar abduction is movement of the thumb in a plane perpendicular to the plane of the palm.

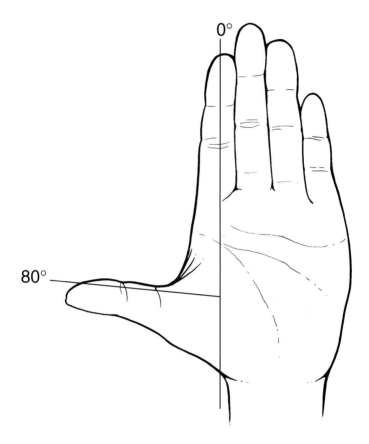

Fig. 8.2   **RADIAL ABDUCTION:** Motion of the thumb parallel to the plane of the palm and away from the radial side of the hand. Palmar abduction is generally greater than radial abduction.

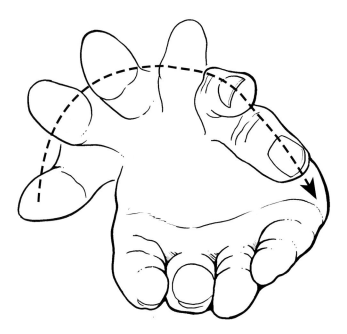

Fig. 8.3   **MOVEMENT OF OPPOSITION**

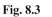

Opposition

Opposition is a composite motion consisting of three elements:
(1) palmar abduction that then progresses to adduction at the
carpometacarpal (CMC) joint, (2) rotation at the CMC joint,
(3) flexion at the CMC, MP, and IP joints of the thumb (Fig. 8.3).
Opposition is valued as 50% to 60% of thumb function[7,42] and
opposition is usually considered complete when the tip of the
thumb touches the base of the fifth finger. A lack of opposition
can be measured as the distance from the tip of the thumb to
the base of the little finger (Fig. 8.4).

Opposition can also be measured as the largest possible span
from the flexor crease of the thumb IP joint to the distal palmar
crease over the third metacarpal (Fig. 8.5). A span of less than
8 cm is considered abnormal.[7,42]

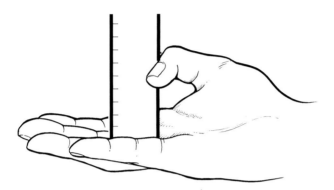

Fig. 8.4   **METHOD OF MEASURING IMPAIRMENT OF OPPOSITION**

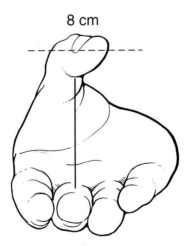

8 cm

Fig. 8.5   **ALTERNATIVE METHOD FOR MEASURING IMPAIRMENT OF THUMB OPPOSITION**

Flexion/Extension

All joints of the thumb move in the plane of flexion-extension (Fig. 8.6). At the thumb CMC joint, this plane of movement is difficult to quantify and, therefore, is rarely measured.

Flexion at the thumb MP (Fig. 8.7) joint can be quite variable. In a study of young adult males, 15% of the subjects had a limited arc of flexion that averaged 27°.[43] The remaining 85% had an arc of thumb MP flexion that averaged 56°. Extension is usually not observed at the thumb MP joint.

Flexion at the IP joint (Fig. 8.8) averaged 73° in a study of young adult males[43] but was 65° ± 12.1° in a report that examined 348 male and female adults ranging in age from 16 to 86 years.[20] Slight extension is commonly seen at the thumb IP joint and averaged 5° in the study of young adult males.[43]

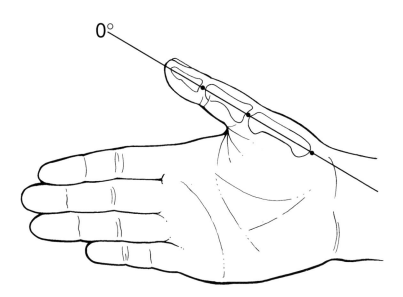

Fig. 8.6   **ZERO STARTING POSITION:** The thumb is extended with the proximal and distal phalanx in line with the thumb metacarpal. The wrist should be maintained in a neutral position. If the wrist is flexed, the extensor pollicis longus will be effectively tenodesed, thereby limiting flexion of the thumb MP and IP joints.

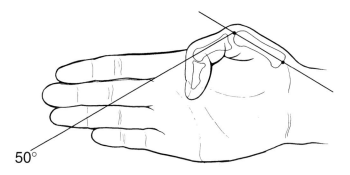

50°

Fig. 8.7   **THUMB METACARPOPHALANGEAL JOINT:**
Flexion 0° to 50°.

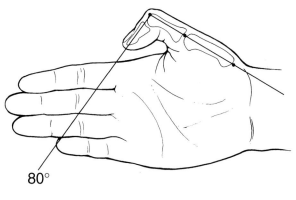

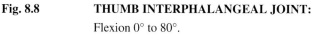

80°

Fig. 8.8   **THUMB INTERPHALANGEAL JOINT:**
Flexion 0° to 80°.

The Cervical Spine

Motion of the cervical spine includes flexion-extension, right and left lateral bending, and right and left rotation. In a radiographic study, Johnson and associates[44] noted that flexion of the cervical spine (mean = 68.6°) was equivalent to extension (mean = 67.9°). Therefore, the cervical spine is unique in that opposite motions are approximately equal, eg, flexion = extension, right rotation = left rotation, and right lateral bending = left lateral bending.

Different vertebral segments, however, do not contribute equivalent amounts to each plane of motion. This is evident for rotation at the C1-C2 level, which accounts for 55% to 60% of cervical rotation.[45,46]

Flexion is limited at the occipit-C1 joint, averaging only 3.5° compared to 21.0° of extension at this vertebral level.[47] From C1 to C6, the range of flexion and the range of extension are approximately equal at each vertebral level.[44] The total arc of flexion-extension is greater in the lower cervical vertebral segments with peak motion occurring at the C5-C6 level.[44,48] The range of flexion is greater than extension from C6 to T1, the difference being most marked at the C7-T1 level.[44]

Rotation of the cervical spine is coupled with lateral bending and flexion-extension. In the lower cervical spine, lateral bending goes in the same direction as rotation and, with maximum rotation to one side, averaged 19.1° for C3 to C7.[49] In the upper cervical spine, lateral bending goes in the direction opposite to rotation, and averaged 4.0° from the occipit to C3. Flexion from the occipit to C5 accompanies rotation (mean flexion = 19.2° at maximum rotation) while extension is coupled with rotation at the C5 to C7 levels (mean = 4.6°).[49]

Lateral bending is also accompanied by rotation. In a study using electric goniometers, lateral bending to one side averaged 46° ± 6.5° and was accompanied by an average rotation of 24° ± 13°.[50]

The normal passive range of cervical spine motion is listed in Table 9.1. The study by Dvorak and associates[22] obtained precise measurements on 150 asymptomatic adults and confirmed clinical impressions that cervical spine motion decreased with age. Decreased motion occurred sooner and was more severe in males.

TABLE 9.1

PASSIVE RANGE OF CERVICAL SPINE MOTION
IN HEALTHY ADULTS[*]

Age	Flexion/Extension	Lateral Bending	Axial Rotation
20-29	$151° \pm 17°$	$101° \pm 11°$	$183° \pm 11°$
30-49	$141° \pm 35°$	$93° \pm 13°$	$172° \pm 13°$
> 50	$129° \pm 14°$	$80° \pm 17°$	$155° \pm 15°$

[*]Adapted from Dvorak and associates.[22] Precise measurements made on 150 asymptomatic adults using CA 6000 Spine Motion Analyzer.

It should be noted that PROM in the cervical spine is consistently greater than AROM, even in asymptomatic subjects.[48,51]

Patients with cervical spine disorders also demonstrate decreased motion in the involved segments. Dvorak and associates[51] measured segmental motion on flexion-extension radiographs in patients with degenerative, radicular, and whiplash trauma disorders. All groups had decreased flexion in the involved segments. The whiplash trauma group had less reduction of motion in the involved segment and also demon-strated a trend toward increased motion in the uninvolved upper and middle cervical regions.

Clinical assessment of cervical spine motion provides an index to the severity of the disorder but is only a composite measure-ment of movement that is occurring throughout the entire neck. On the other hand, specialized radiographic techniques used for research purposes are costly, complex, and unnecessary for most clinical situations. Routine radiographs can usually identify the cervical vertebrae that are diseased or injured.

Assessment of cervical spine motion is usually based on visual estimation (Figs. 9.1-9.3). The prominent midline position of the nose and chin makes visual estimation relatively accurate. The routine use of a goniometer in measuring cervical spine motion is somewhat cumbersome but when used in a very stan-dardized fashion, measurement with a goniometer can be more reliable than visual estimation.[52] Inclinometers can also be used to measure cervical spine motion. In a study by Alund and Larsson,[50] the inclinometer showed good correlation coeffi-cients for measuring flexion-extension and lateral bending, but poor correlation when measuring rotation.

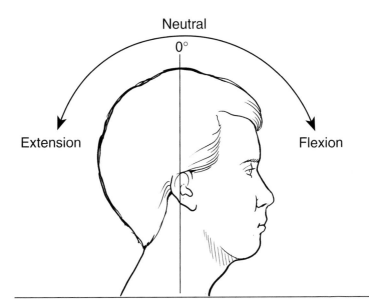

Fig. 9.1   **FLEXION AND EXTENSION:**
ZERO STARTING POSITION.

The neck is aligned with the trunk. Flexion is forward bending of the cervical spine, while extension is posterior inclination of the neck. It is important to stabilize the trunk so that
motion is not occurring in the thoracic spine. These motions
are usually designated in degrees; however, limited flexion
may also be measured as the distance the chin lacks in touching the sternum.

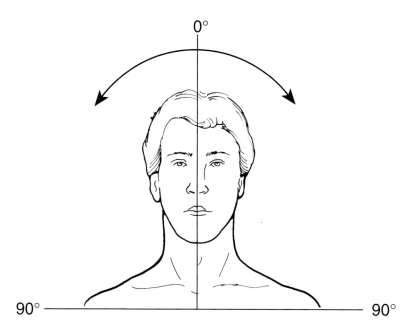

Fig. 9.2   **LATERAL BEND: ZERO STARTING POSITION.**
The nose is vertical and perpendicular to the axis of the
shoulders. It is important to stabilize the trunk so that motion
occurs only at the neck. Right lateral bend is with the head
deviated toward the right, and left lateral bend is the opposite
direction. The degree of lateral bend is determined by the
angle between the mid axis of the face and the vertical.

The Clinical Measurement of Joint Motion

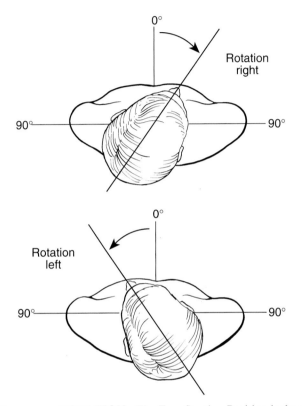

Fig. 9.3　　　　**ROTATION:** The Zero Starting Position is the same as for measuring lateral bend. Right rotation is with the head turned to the right, and left rotation is with the head turned to the left. Rotation is estimated in degrees from the Zero Starting Position. Positioning the cervical spine in maximum flexion essentially eliminates rotation from occurring in the lower cervical vertebrae. Measuring rotation in this position, therefore, will assess the degree of rotation occurring in the upper cervical vertebrae.[22]

The Thoracic and Lumbar Spine

As in the cervical spine, thoracic and lumbar spine motion is a composite measurement of several joints. The planes of motion are also similar; ie, flexion/extension, right and left lateral bend, and right and left rotation. Decreased motion is also observed in older adults.[53-57]

Radiographic studies analyzing segmental motion are helpful in understanding normal kinematics of the lumbar spine. Those outlined in Table 10.1 are in vivo studies on asymptomatic young to middle-age adults. Furthermore, these studies used dynamic radiographs made in the standing position, an important technical point, because maximal lumbar flexion cannot be achieved when the patient is sitting.[58]

Greater arcs of motion were recorded in the study by Dvorak and associates,[58] who measured passive range of motion, whereas Pearcy and associates[59,60] used active, voluntary movement (Table 10.1). This difference in technique may explain the different range of motion in the two studies, as passive motion of the lumbar spine has been shown to be greater than active motion.[61]

TABLE 10.1

RADIOGRAPHIC ANALYSIS OF LUMBAR SPINE MOTION IN ASYMPTOMATIC ADULTS

Vertebral Segment	Flexion/Extension		Lateral (right to left) Bending		Rotation (right to left total)
	Dvorak, et al [58]	Pearcy, et al [59]	Dvorak, et al [58]	Pearcy, et al [60]	Pearcy, et al [60]
L1-L2	11.9° ± 2.3°*	13° ± 5°**	10.4° ± 2.8°*	10° **	2°**
L2-L3	14.5° ± 2.3°	14° ± 2°	12.4° ± 3.4°	11°	2°
L3-L4	15.3° ± 2.0°	13° ± 2°	12.4° ± 4.3°	10°	3°
L4-L5	18.2° ± 3.0°	16° ± 4°	9.5° ± 4.9°	6°	3°
L5-S1	17.0° ± 4.3°	14° ± 5°	5.1°**	3°	2°
TOTAL	76.9°	70°	49.8°	40°	12°

* Average ± standard deviation
** Standard deviation not provided.

The salient points concerning lumbar spine motion are that flexion/extension is greatest in the lower lumbar segments, while lateral bending is most limited at the lumbosacral junction (Table 10.1). The arcs of rotational movements are relatively small throughout the lumbar spine.

Limited information is available concerning normal kinematics of the thoracic spine, as the overlying ribs do not permit dynamic radiographic studies. Gregersen and Lucas[62] drilled pins into selected spinous processes of seven male volunteers, but in only one subject could rotation be measured throughout the thoracic spine. In this subject, rotation in the standing position was 70° as measured from T1 to T12. White[63] made detailed measurements of segmental motion on 10 autopsy specimens after applying various loads. The range of flexion/extension gradually increased from the upper thoracic to the lower thoracic segments with the arc of motion being particularly large at the T10-T11 and T11-T12 interspace. By contrast, the greatest amount of axial rotation occurred in the upper thoracic spine. The arc of lateral bending was relatively constant throughout the thoracic spine but did show a slight increase in the lower thoracic segments. White and Panjabi[64] listed 63° as a representative arc of flexion/extension in the thoracic spine and segmental motion ranging from 4° at the T1-T2 interspace to 12° at the T11-T12 interspace. A representative arc of axial rotation to one side was 62°, being 9° at the T1-T2 interspace compared with only 2° at the T11-T12 interspace. A representative range of lateral bending to one side was 68°, being 5° at the T1-T2 interspace and 9° at the T11-T12 interspace.

Standard methods of measuring joint motion are difficult to apply in the thoracic and lumbar spine. Therefore, some clinicians question the value of measuring spine motion. Alternative methods of measurement have been devised and advocated, but without agreement about which method is best.

Methods of assessing thoracic and lumbar spine motion can be classified as visual estimation, goniometric measurements, skin distraction, and inclinometer techniques. Because prominent midline landmarks are not easily seen, visual estimation can provide only a subjective impression of thoracic and lumbar spine motion. Likewise, the extensive soft tissue coverage makes goniometric measurements difficult. Skin distraction and inclinometer techniques provide a more objective and reproducible assessment of motion in this region.

With movement, skin distracts or attracts over the joint(s). Skin distraction can be easily measured with a tape measure, a tool that is readily available. The change in distance reflects the degree of motion. Tape measure techniques, however, cannot assess rotation, are affected by the patient's size, and do not measure motion in degrees.

The double inclinometer method measures spine motion in degrees, is not affected by the patient's height or skin elasticity, and can measure all planes of motion. This technique of measurement takes longer to perform,[65] and inclinometers are not readily available. In addition, some studies of lumbar spine motion have found that skin distraction measurements are more reliable than the double inclinometer technique.[65,66]

Various techniques of measuring thoracic and lumbar spine motion will be described. Methods utilizing a tape measure are appropriate for most clinical examinations. The normal range of motion for selected techniques is listed in Table 10.2 (p. 98). An inclinometer may be the technique of choice for disability ratings that require this method[7] or when one is doing clinical research that needs comparative measurements recorded in degrees.

Flexion

Zero Starting Position (Figure 10.1)

The subject stands with the hips and knees straight and the trunk in line with the lower extremities. The feet should be comfortably

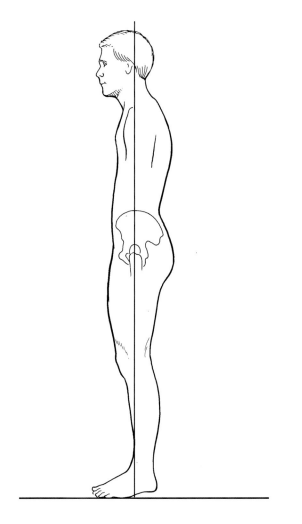

Fig. 10.1   **ZERO STARTING POSITION**

apart to facilitate movement of the spine. The arms normally hang in a relaxed, extended position.

Visual Estimation

Sagittal alignment of the lumbar spine changes during flexion, ie, the normal lumbar lordosis is lost. An asymptomatic lumbar spine will actually go into slight kyphosis during flexion (Fig. 10.2). The angle of trunk inclination from the Zero Starting Position can be estimated. Because a large segment of this movement is occurring at the hips, any restriction of hip flexion will limit forward inclination of the trunk and visual assessment of spine motion. In a similar fashion, contractures of the hamstrings will also restrict forward bending of the spine.

At maximum flexion, the distance between the fingertips and the floor should be visualized and can be measured. The fingertip-to-floor method, however, has poor repeatability[65] and is not a reliable method for following a patient with a low back problem.

Skin Distraction (Thoracic and Lumbar Flexion)

With the patient standing in the Zero Starting Position, the spinous processes of T1 and S1 are marked (Fig. 10.3). As the patient flexes the trunk, the skin will distract. The distance between T1 and S1 is again measured with the patient inclined

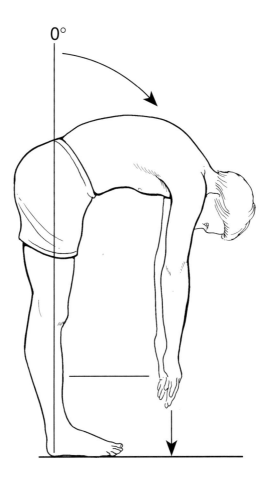

0°

Fig. 10.2   **VISUAL ESTIMATION OF THORACIC AND LUMBAR SPINE FLEXION**

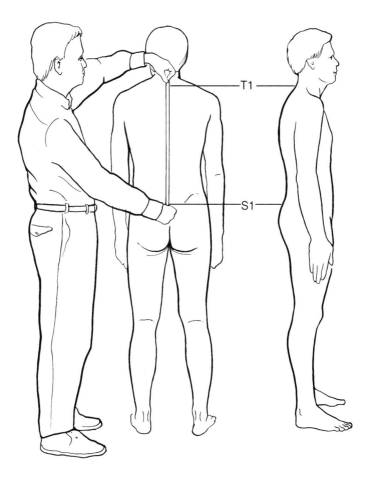

Fig. 10.3   **SKIN DISTRACTION MEASUREMENT OF
THORACIC AND LUMBAR FLEXION:
ZERO STARTING POSITION**

forward in maximum flexion (Fig. 10.4). A typical measurement will be > 10 cm, but, to our knowledge, there are no reported normal values for this method of measurement. This measurement is uncommonly performed, as it does not isolate lumbar spine movement.

Modified Schober Test (Lumbar Flexion)

Schober[67] initially described a technique of measuring skin distraction to assess lumbar flexion, but the modified Schober test described by Macrae and Wright[68] in 1969 has achieved common usage. The modified Schober test is performed by making a midline mark on a line connecting the dimples of Venus (indicates the lower half of the posterior superior iliac spine). Macrae and Wright[68] originally described this mark as overlying the lumbosacral junction, but a line connecting the posterior superior iliac spine actually intersects the second sacral segment.[69] The skin is then marked 5 cm below and 10 cm above the first point (Fig. 10.5). After the patient inclines into maximum flexion, the distance between the upper and lower points is again measured. The increased length of the measurement, ie, the distance > 15 cm, is recorded as the degree of lumbar flexion.

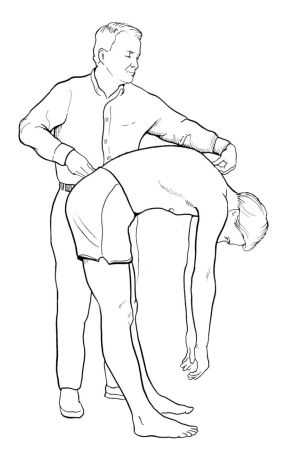

Fig. 10.4   **RECORDING FLEXION:** The amount of flexion is
recorded as the distance from T1 to S1 in the Zero Starting
Position subtracted from the distance measured with the
subject inclined into maximum flexion.

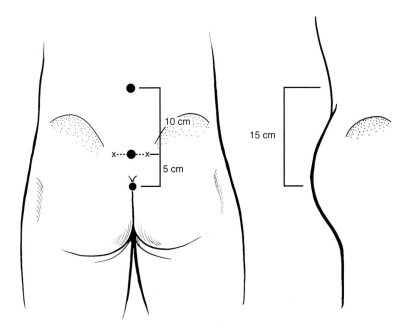

Fig. 10.5   **MODIFIED SCHOBER TEST:**
ZERO STARTING POSITION.
A 15-cm span is measured from 10 cm above a line
connecting the posterior superior iliac spine (PSIS) to 5 cm
below this line.

The modified Schober test (Fig. 10.6) in asymptomatic adults averaged 6.3 cm in the study by Macrae and Wright[68] and 6.9 cm in the study by Battie and associates.[23] Normal values for adult males and females of various ages have also been determined (Table 10.2).

The advantage of the modified Schober method is that there are values for comparison.[53,68] Furthermore, clinical studies have shown satisfactory intrarater and interrater reliability for this technique.[53,54] Gill and associates[66] also observed better relia-bility with the modified Schober test compared with the double inclinometer technique.

The disadvantage of the modified Schober test is that by going 5 cm below the posterior superior iliac spine (PSIS), the immobile lower sacrum and coccyx are included in the measurement parameters. In addition, Miller and associates[70] noted that a mark 10 cm above the PSIS ranged from the L-1 spinous process to the L3-L4 interspace with the median point being the L2-L3 interspace. Therefore, in adults, the modified Schober test includes too much skin distraction over the immobile sacrum and does not measure skin distraction over the entire lumbar spine.

The Clinical Measurement of Joint Motion

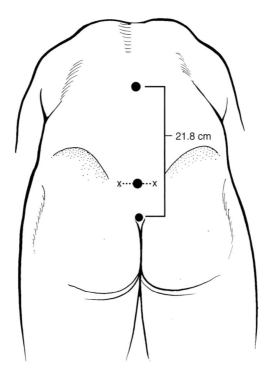

Fig. 10.6   **MODIFIED SCHOBER TEST:**
The number recorded is the distance on maximum flexion
minus 15 cm. In this subject, 6.8 cm would be listed as the
degree of flexion.

Simplified Skin Distraction Measurement of Lumbar Flexion

Van Adrichem and van der Korst[71] studied skin distraction during lumbar flexion at points made 5, 10, 15, and 20 cm above the PSIS. Limited distraction was observed between the 15- and 20-centimeter mark. Therefore, these authors advocated measuring lumbar flexion between two midline points: one made at the level of the PSIS and the second made 15 cm higher (Fig. 10.7). In a group of 15- to 18-year-old subjects, the simplified skin distraction technique averaged 6.7 ± 1.0 cm in males and 5.8 ± 0.9 cm in females.[71]

This method of measuring lumbar flexion is simpler than the modified Schober test. Furthermore, the lower sacrum is not included in this measurement and a mark 15 cm above the PSIS should encompass the entire lumbar spine in adult subjects.

This simplified skin distraction method has also been compared with the double inclinometer method in a group of patients with chronic low back pain.[65] Better intratester and better intertester reliability was observed with the simplified skin distraction technique. The disadvantage of this method is that normal values for all ages have not been determined.

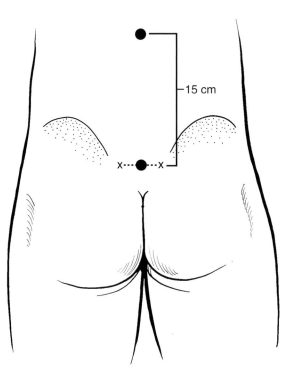

15 cm

Fig. 10.7   **SIMPLIFIED SKIN DISTRACTION MEASUREMENT OF LUMBAR FLEXION:** With the patient in the Zero Starting Position, a 15-cm span is measured from a line connecting the posterior superior iliac spines. The distance between these endpoints is remeasured with the patient in maximum flexion. The degree of flexion is the distance between these points on maximum flexion minus 15 cm.

Double Inclinometer Method—Lumbar Flexion

In 1967, Loebl[55] described measurement of lumbar spine flexion with two inclinometers. Recent studies by Mayer and associates[72] and others[73-75] have renewed interest in this technique. With the patient standing in the Zero Starting Position (Fig. 10.8A), one inclinometer is placed over the sacrum and the second is positioned over the T12 spinous process. The dials of the inclinometers are set at zero. The patient then leans forward into maximum flexion (Fig. 10.8B). The degree of inclination on the sacral inclinometer represents flexion of the hip, while the reading on the T12 inclinometer represents total body flexion. To calculate lumbar flexion, the degrees recorded with the sacral inclinometer are subtracted from the degrees recorded on the T12 inclinometer.

The degree of lumbar flexion at different ages as measured by the inclinometer technique is listed in Table 10.2. In young adults, the total arc of flexion/extension averaged 107° in the study by Loebl[55] and 92° in the study by Keeley and associates.[73] This range of motion is higher than that observed in radiographic studies,[58,59] and the discrepancy is of concern. Furthermore, no study has analyzed the consistency of positioning the inclinometer over the T12 interspace.

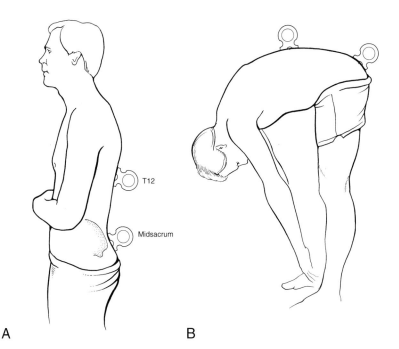

A   B

Fig. 10.8A   **DOUBLE INCLINOMETER METHOD:**
                  ZERO STARTING POSITION.
                  The inclinometers are aligned over T12 and the sacrum and
                  their gauges are set at 0°.

Fig. 10.8B   The subject positions the spine in maximum flexion. The
                  degrees recorded on the sacral inclinometer are subtracted
                  from the degrees recorded on the inclinometer positioned
                  over the T12 spinous process.

Therefore, skin distraction techniques, and specifically, the simplified skin distraction method seem preferable when measuring lumbar flexion.

Double Inclinometer Method—Thoracic Flexion

To measure flexion of the thoracic spine, the patient assumes the Zero Starting Position in either a sitting or standing position. The inclinometers are aligned in the sagittal plane over the spinous process of T1 and T12. Both inclinometers are set to zero. The patient is asked to lean forward into a position of maximum thoracic flexion. The degree of thoracic flexion is obtained by subtracting the T12 inclinometer reading from the T1 inclinometer reading. Extension of the thoracic spine is limited and, therefore, is usually not measured.

Extension

Visual Method

The subject places the palms on the buttocks while standing in the Zero Starting Position. The patient is then asked to lean back as far as possible. Extension of the spine can be visually estimated. An approximate measurement can also be obtained with a goniometer.[53,54]

Skin Attraction—Modified Schober

Skin attraction has been used to assess lumbar extension. Beattie and associates[76] used the same landmarks developed for the modified Schober test. The decreased distance after maximal extension of the spine was subtracted from the starting distance of 15 cm (eg, 15 cm - 12.5 cm = 2.5 cm of lumbar extension). In 100 asymptomatic adults, mean extension was 1.6 ± 0.7 cm.[76] Intratester and intertester reliability was satisfactory. The objections to using these landmarks for measuring extension of the lumbar spine would be the same as those described for the modified Schober method of measuring lumbar flexion.

Simplified Skin Attraction Measurement of Lumbar Extension

Lumbar spine extension also can be measured using a midline point at the level of the posterior superior iliac spine and a midline mark 15 cm superior to the PSIS (Fig. 10.9). Williams and associates[65] compared the simplified skin attraction method to the double inclinometer method in patients with chronic low back pain. Simplified skin attraction method had better reliability.

The advantages of the simplified skin attraction tests for measuring lumbar extension are the same as those listed for lumbar

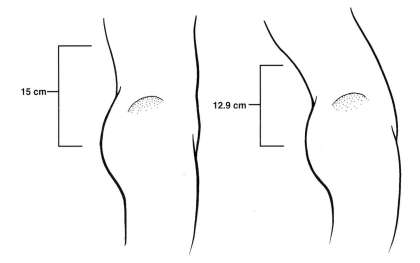

Fig. 10.9 **SIMPLIFIED SKIN ATTRACTION MEASUREMENT OF LUMBAR EXTENSION.:** A 15-cm span is marked as described in Fig. 10.7. The patient places the spine in maximum extension. The value recorded is 15 cm minus the distance measured in maximum extension.

In this patient, lumbar extension would be recorded as 2.1 cm.

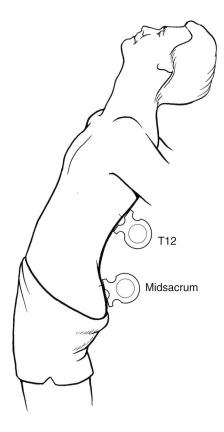

T12

Midsacrum

Fig. 10.10   **EXTENSION: DOUBLE INCLINOMETER METHOD.**
The range of extension is recorded in degrees by subtracting
the measurement in the sacrum indicated from the reading on
the inclinometer placed over T12.

flexion. The disadvantages of this method are that normal values are not available for comparison.

Double Inclinometer Method

The Starting Position and placement of the inclinometers are the same as those used in measuring flexion of the lumbar spine. After the patient extends maximally, the degree of inclination on each instrument is recorded (Fig. 10.10). Lumbar extension is obtained by subtracting the degree of pelvic extension (determined by the inclinometer over the sacrum) from the total arc of extension (obtained from the reading on the inclinometer over the T12 spinous process). In 28 normal adult subjects, lumbar spine extension averaged 27 ± 9.6° when measured by inclinometers.[73]

Lateral Bending

Visual Estimation and Goniometric Measurement

With the patient in the Zero Starting Position, the T1, T12, and S1 spinous processes are marked. To measure right lateral bending, the patient laterally inclines the trunk to the right while keeping the knees straight. Lateral bend of the spine can be visually estimated, or an approximate measurement can be obtained with a goniometer.[53,54]

Tape Measure Method

Skin attraction methods have been described for measuring lateral bend of the lumbar spine[57] but are somewhat difficult to apply. Mellin[77] described a tape measure technique that is easy to perform. With the patient in the Zero Starting Position, a point is marked on the leg at the tip of the long finger (Fig. 10.11). The patient then laterally inclines the spine and a second mark is made on the leg at the tip of the long finger. The distance between the two points is the measurement of thoracic and lumbar lateral bend.

In 39 asymptomatic subjects, lateral bending of the spine averaged 21.6 ± 5.4 cm by this technique.[77] In 476 patients with low back pain, tape measurement of lateral bend demonstrated better correlation with the degree of disability than inclinometer measurements.[77]

Double Inclinometer Method

The inclinometers are positioned over the sacrum and the T12 spinous process with the patient in the Zero Starting Position. To measure right lateral bend of the lumbar spine, the patient bends the trunk maximally to the right and the angles on both inclinometers are recorded. Right lateral bend is calculated by subtracting sacral inclination from the T12 inclinometer read-

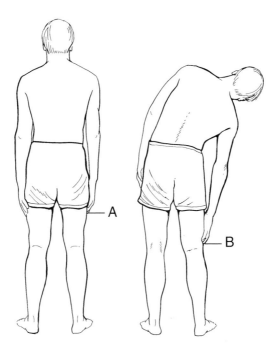

Fig. 10.11A, B   **TAPE MEASUREMENT OF LATERAL BEND:**
(A) The thigh is marked at the tip of the long finger with the
patient in the Zero Starting Position and (B) with the spine
positioned in maximum lateral bend. The distance between
the two positions is the value recorded for lateral bend.

ing. To determine left lateral bend of the lumbar spine, the process is repeated with the patient inclining maximally in a left lateral direction.

Spine Rotation

Visual Method

To estimate the degree of spinal rotation, the pelvis must be held firmly by the examiner's hands. The patient is instructed to rotate to the right and then to the left while maintaining the scapula in a neutral position. The motion is estimated in degrees based on a line drawn through the plane of the shoulders (Fig. 10.12).

Double-Inclinometer Method

To measure rotation of the thoracic spine, the patient flexes the spine until the trunk is parallel to the floor. Inclinometers are positioned over the T1 and T12 spinous processes and set at 0 (Fig. 10.13A). The patient then rotates the trunk maximally to the left while keeping the arms folded in a position to minimize shoulder motion (Fig. 10.13B). The degree of thoracic rotation is the T12 inclinometer angle subtracted from the T1 angle. Rotation should be at least 30° to each side, ie, 60° total arc of rotation.[7]

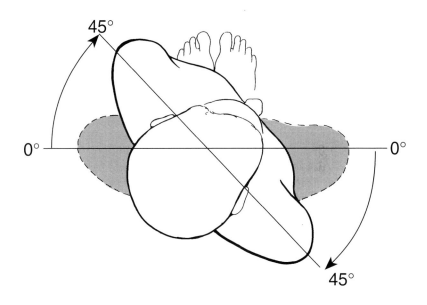

Fig. 10.12 **VISUAL ESTIMATION OF SPINAL ROTATION**

The Clinical Measurement of Joint Motion

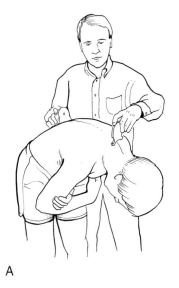 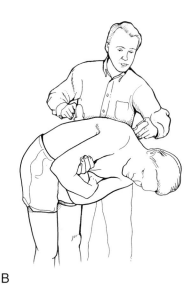

A   B

Fig. 10.13A   Zero starting position for double inclinometer method of measuring thoracic rotation.

Fig. 10.13B   Spine is positioned in maximum rotation to the left. The neck should be maintained in a neutral position.

Rotation of the lumbar spine can be measured in a similar fashion with inclinometers placed over the T12 spinous processes and the sacrum. In a limited study of 12 normal subjects, rotation of the lumbar spine averaged 21 ± 3.3°.[73] When using the double inclinometer technique, Boline[78] found less rotation in asymptomatic subjects compared to those with low back pain; however, errors in prediction and examiner disagreement were relatively large compared to the scale of measurement.

TABLE 10.2

CLINICAL MEASUREMENTS OF LUMBAR SPINE MOTION

Age/Gender	Flexion: Modified Schober[a] (cm ± s.d.)	Flexion: Simplified Skin Distraction[b] (cm ± s.d.)	Flexion: Inclinometer[c] (degrees)	Extension: Modified Schober[d] (cm)	Extension: Inclinometer[c] (degrees)	Lateral Bend: Goniometer[e] (degrees)
Young Adult Male	7.4 ± 0.9	6.7 ± 1.0	66	1.9	38	38 ± 5.8
Middle Aged Male	7.0 ± 1.0		58	1.2	35	29 ± 6.5
Older Aged Male	5.5 ± 1.3		49		33	19 ± 4.8
Young Adult Female	6.7 ± 1.1	5.8 ± 0.9	67	1.8	42	35 ± 6.4
Middle Aged Female	6.1 ± 1.2		60	1.4	40	30 ± 5.8
Older Aged Female	5.0 ± 1.0		44		36	23 ± 5.4

a   Adapted with permission from[49]. In this study, young adult was 15-34 years old, middle age was 35-64 years old, and older adult was ≥ 65 years.

b   Adapted with permission from[79]. Young adult was 15-18 years old.

c   Adapted with permission from[55]. In this study, young adult was 15-30 years old, middle age was 31-60 years old, and older aged was ≥ 61 years.

d   Adapted with permission from[76]. In this study, young adult was 16-28 years old, middle age was 29-57 years old.

e   Adapted with permission from[54] for males and adapted with permission from[53] for females.
    In this study, young adult was 20-29 years, middle age adult was 30-59 years, and older adult was 60-84 years.

The Hip

The hip is a ball and socket joint capable of considerable triaxial motion. The acetabulum, in comparison to the glenoid, is considerably deeper and, therefore, the range of hip motion is considerably less than the shoulder, the other ball and socket joint.

Normal range of hip motion at different ages is listed in Table 11.1. The data included in this table are from studies that measured hip motion using methods described in this chapter.

Hip motion is strikingly different in newborn children. Many studies have confirmed that neonates have a significant hip flexion contracture that averaged 28° in the study by Haas and associates,[79] 30° in the study by Forero and associates,[26] 46° in the study by Waugh and associates,[80] and ranged from 50° to 80° in the report by Hoffer.[27] Neonates have more external rotation than internal rotation.[23,26,79] The total arc of hip rotation is also increased, averaging 171° in neonates[26] compared with the 90° to 100° arc of rotation normally seen in children older than one year of age. Because rotation is greater with the hip in flexion, the increased range of hip rotation in neonates may be secondary to their associated flexion contracture.

The hip flexion contracture and excessive hip external rotation gradually resolve over the first year of life.[28,81] By the age of 2 years, the mean internal and external rotation are approximately equal;[29,81] however, any individual child or adult may demonstrate a relatively greater degree of internal or external rotation. Excessive femoral anteversion, a common cause of intoeing in children, is characterized by increased internal rotation and limited external rotation of the hip.

The range of hip motion is generally greater in children than in adults (Table 11.1). Adults, however, demonstrate very little decline in hip motion with advancing age. In a study of 1,683 healthy adults, Roach and Miles[24] found minimal change in hip motion up to the age of 74 years. They concluded that any substantial loss of joint mobility should be viewed as abnormal and not attributable to aging.

Hip motion is best measured with the patient lying either supine or prone. Errors in measurement will occur if the examiner fails to recognize tilt or rotation of the pelvis (Figs. 11.1–11.13).

Measurement of hip extension has the greatest variability on a percentage basis (Table 11.1). Obtaining this measurement while maintaining neutral pelvic alignment is cumbersome and awkward, particularly in an adult. In most clinical situations, whether or not a patient has hip extension is not significant. Therefore, many clinicians do not measure extension when examining the hip. Of more importance is whether or not the hip has a flexion contracture.

Rotation can be measured with the hip in extension or flexion. Extension is preferred in most situations, as that position approximates the functional posture of the hip during walking and most other upright activities. Furthermore, with the hip in flexion, the capsular structures are relaxed, and the arc of rotation, particularly in the external plane, is much greater. Measurement of rotation with the hip flexed is preferred in elderly patients and in others whose medical problems do not permit prone positioning. Patients who are suspected of having slipped capital femoral epiphysis should also have their rotation measured with the hip flexed. This is the one deformity in which internal rotation is less when the hip is flexed than when it is extended.

Table 11.1

HIP MOTION AT DIFFERENT AGES (IN DEGREES)

	Neonate[26] Mean±s.d.	4 Year[19] Mean±2s.d.	8 Year[19] Mean±2s.d.	11 Year[19] Mean±2s.d.	Adult[14] Mean±s.d.	Adult[24] Mean±s.d.	Adult[18] Mean±s.d.
Extension	minus 30±3.9	29±6.3	27±6.3	25±14.0	12±5.4	19±8	9± 5.2
Flexion	128±4.8	150±12.5	146±11.3	138±14.5	121±6.4	121±13	120±8.3
Abduction	79*±4.3	54±9.0	49±7.3	45±10.8	41±6.0	42±11	39±7.2
Adduction	17±3.5	30±5.0	28±6.0	29±6.3	27±3.6	—	31±7.3
Internal Rotation	76±5.6	55±17.8	54±17.5	48±16.0	44±4.3	32±8	33±8.2
External Rotation	92±3.0	46±16.8	43±17.5	42±15.3	44±4.8	32±9	34±6.8

* Measured in flexion. Other studies in adults and older children measured abduction with hip extended (in neutral).

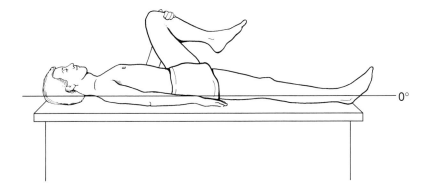

0°

Fig. 11.1   **FLEXION:**
ZERO STARTING POSITION OF THE RIGHT HIP.
The patient lies supine on a firm, flat surface with the
opposite hip held in enough flexion to flatten the lumbar
spine. Flattening the lumbar spine prevents excessive lordosis that can camouflage a hip flexion contracture. On the
other hand, positioning the opposite hip in excessive flexion will rock the pelvis into an abnormal degree of posteri-
or inclination, thereby creating a false positive hip flexion
deformity. The opposite hip should be flexed to a position
where the lumbar spine just starts to flatten or, more pre-
cisely, to a position where the inclination of the anterior
superior iliac spine (ASIS) is similar to a normal standing
posture; ie, the ASIS is inferior to the PSIS by only two to
three degrees.

The Clinical Measurement of Joint Motion

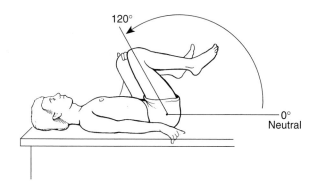

Fig. 11.2   **MAXIMUM FLEXION:**

Maximum flexion is the point where the pelvis begins to rotate. Flexion for this subject is recorded from 0° to 120°.

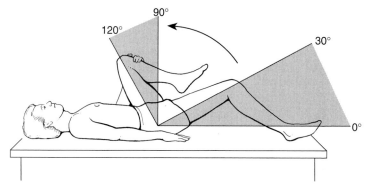

Fig. 11.3   **LIMITED MOTION IN FLEXION:**

Limited motion (unshaded area) is noted as in the elbow and knee.

(1) The hip flexes from 30° to 90° (30°→ 90°).

(2) The hip has a flexion deformity or flexion contracture of 30° with further flexion to 90° (30° FC W/ FF 90°).

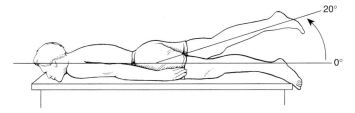

Fig. 11.4A   **EXTENSION: ZERO STARTING POSITION.**
The patient lies prone on a firm level surface. The leg is
extended with the knee either straight or flexed. Maximum
extension is recorded when the pelvis starts to rotate.

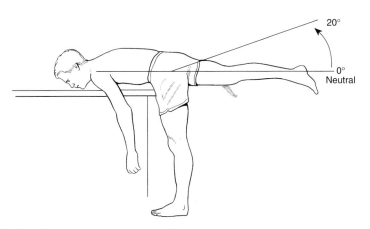

Fig. 11.4B   Another method flexes the opposite extremity over the end of
the examination table. Movement of the pelvis is more easily
ascertained in this position. This method, however, is awkward in an adult but easier to perform in a child. A flexion
contracture of the hip in a child also can be measured in the
prone position. This is particularly useful when a knee flexion
contracture is also present.

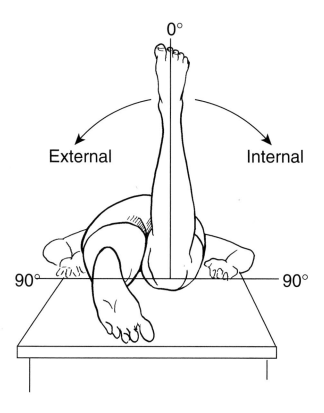

Fig. 11.5   **ROTATION: ZERO STARTING POSITION.**
The patient is prone and the knee flexed to 90°. The axis of
the tibia provides a clear landmark for assessing rotation.

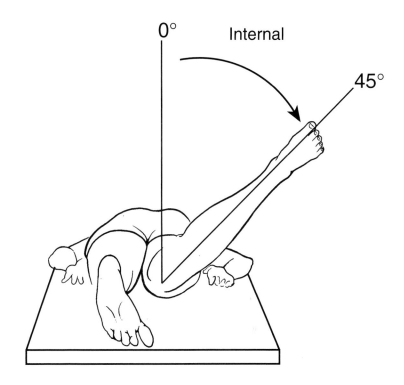

0°   Internal

45°

Fig. 11.6   **INTERNAL ROTATION:** Internal rotation is obtained by
rotating the leg outward, thereby causing the hip to go into
internal rotation. The degree of internal rotation is the angle
that the tibia makes with the Zero Starting Position. By measuring both hips at the same time, neutral alignment of the
pelvis is maintained.

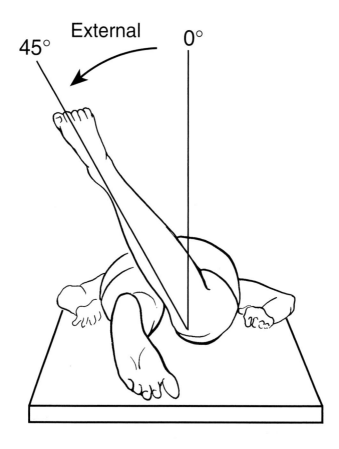

Fig. 11.7 **EXTERNAL ROTATION:** External rotation is measured by rotating the leg inward, thereby externally rotating the hip joint. Maximum external rotation is achieved when the pelvis starts to tilt, a movement that can be ascertained by keeping one hand on the pelvis.

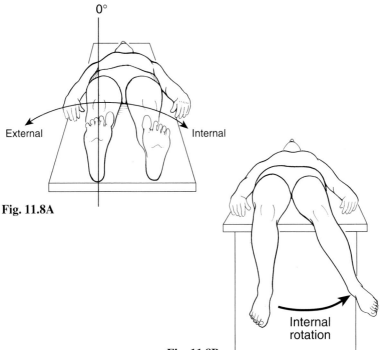

Fig. 11.8A

Fig. 11.8B

Fig. 11.8A   **MEASUREMENT OF ROTATION WITH THE PATIENT SUPINE:** Rotation with the hips extended can also be measured with the patient supine.

Fig. 11.8B   **MEASUREMENT OF ROTATION WITH THE PATIENT SUPINE:** Flexing the knees over the end of the table, if possible, will improve accuracy of measurement.

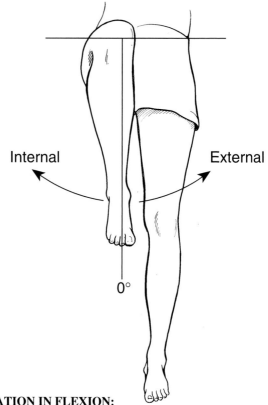

Fig. 11.9   **ROTATION IN FLEXION:**
               ZERO STARTING POSITION.
               With the patient lying supine, the hip and knee are flexed to
               90°. The thigh is perpendicular to the transverse line across
               the anterior superior iliac spines of the pelvis.
               Internal rotation is measured by rotating the tibia away
               from the midline of the trunk, thus producing inward rotation
               of the hip. External rotation is measured by rotating the tibia
               toward the midline of the trunk, thus producing external
               rotation at the hip.

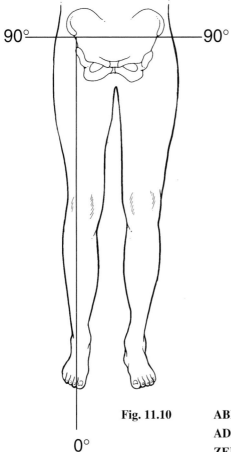

Fig. 11.10

ABDUCTION AND ADDUCTION: ZERO STARTING POSITION.

The patient lies supine with the legs at right angles to a transverse line across the anterior superior iliac spines of the pelvis.

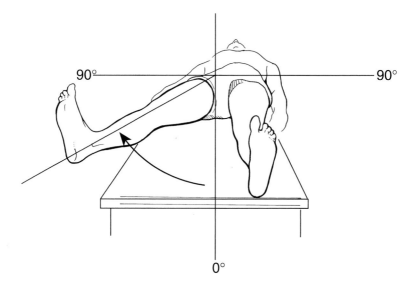

90°   90°

0°

Fig. 11.11   **ABDUCTION:**

Abduction is measured in degrees from the Zero Starting
Position. Maximum abduction is reached when the pelvis
starts to tilt, a movement that can be detected by the examiner keeping his/her hand on the patient's opposite ASIS
when moving the leg.

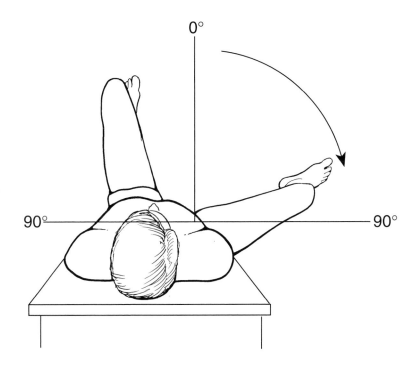

Fig. 11.12   **ABDUCTION IN FLEXION:**
Abduction can also be measured with the hip held in flexion. To enhance repeatability, the hip should be positioned in 90° of flexion. Measuring hip abduction in flexion is particularly useful in neonates and young infants.

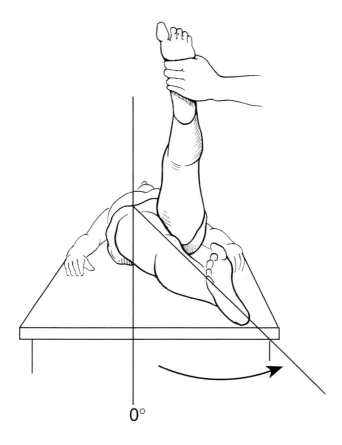

0°

Fig. 11.13   **ADDUCTION:**

The opposite extremity should be elevated to allow adduction, while keeping the hip in the neutral position. Maximum adduction is reached when the pelvis starts to rotate. If elevating the opposite extremity is impractical, the examiner should measure adduction by moving the extremity over the top of the opposite leg.

The Knee

Knee motion is principally flexion and extension. Rotation of the tibia on the femur occurs during movement of the knee, but the degree of rotation is small and cannot be measured accurately.

Knee extension is more often seen in young children. Wynne-Davies,[11] in a study of 3,000 Edinburgh children, noted that 15% of the 3-year-old children could extend their knee beyond 10°, but this degree of extension was observed in < 1% at age 6 years. Cheng and associates[10] noted a greater degree of knee extension in a study of 2,360 Chinese children, but again, extension decreased as the children became older, averaging 16° ± 9° at age 3 compared to a mean of 7° ± 9° by age 10 years. Professional ballet dancers maintain an arc of knee extension,[31] but in most adults, knee extension is not present. Indeed, in two large series of healthy adult males, the average knee extension was a minus 2° ± 3°.[14,18] In essence, it is normal for adults to have a slight flexion contracture at the knee joint.

Knee flexion in healthy adults averaged 141° ± 5.3° in the study by Boone and Azen[14] and 144° ± 6.5° in the study by Roaas and Andersson.[18] As with the hip, the degree of knee flexion shows insignificant changes in older adults.[18]

The technique of measuring flexion and extension in the knee has been described and illustrated in Chapter 1.

The Ankle

Ankle motion is primarily flexion (usually termed dorsiflexion) and extension (usually termed plantar flexion) (Fig. 13.1). As the foot goes from dorsiflexion to plantar flexion, much of the motion occurs at the tibiotalar joint, but other joints from the talonavicular and calcaneocuboid to the tarsometatarsal joints also contribute to dorsiflexion/plantar flexion.[82,83] Therefore, it is not surprising that Backer and Kofoed[84] found that clinical measurements of dorsiflexion/plantar flexion were greater than radiographic measurements of tibiotalar motion.

When performing clinical measurements, it is very difficult, if not impossible, to differentiate motion at the tibiotalar joint from the dorsiflexion/plantar flexion that is occurring at other joints. This differentiation, however, is not critical, as the total arc of plantar flexion and dorsiflexion is more important from a functional standpoint. Therefore, it is understood that clinical measurements of "ankle motion" also record the plantar flexion and dorsiflexion that are occurring at other joints of the hindfoot and midfoot.

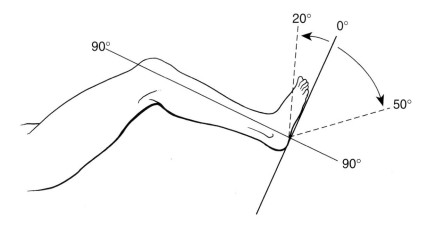

Fig. 13.1   **DORSIFLEXION AND PLANTAR FLEXION:**
The Zero Starting Position is with the knee flexed to relax the heel cord. The foot is perpendicular to the tibia. The goniometer is aligned with the axis of the leg and the lateral side of the plantar surface of the foot. Dorsiflexion (extension) is measured in degrees from the Zero Starting Position when the foot is moved toward the anterior surface of the tibia. Plantar flexion (flexion) is measured in degrees from the Zero Starting Position when the foot is moved away from the anterior surface of the tibia.

Two studies[14,18] analyzed ankle motion in healthy adult males by methods described in *Joint Motion: Method of Measuring and Recording*[33] (Table 13.1). The average arc of motion was 14° greater in the study by Boone and Azen,[14] who measured active range of motion. Roaas and Andersson,[18] however, assessed ankle motion by passive techniques. Using precise landmarks and photographic measurements, Bohannon and associates[85] also demonstrated that ankle motion by active assisted movement was significantly increased compared with passive motion. Therefore, when measuring ankle motion, it is important to note whether one is measuring active or passive range of motion.

TABLE 13.1

ANKLE RANGE OF MOTION IN HEALTHY ADULT MALES

	Boone and Azen[14] (Mean ± s.d.)	Roaas and Andersson[18] (Mean ± s.d.)
Dorsiflexion	13° ± 4.4°	15° ± 5.8°
Plantar Flexion	56° ± 6.1°	40° ± 7.5°

Age and gender also affect ankle motion. Nigg and associates[86] used a specially constructed frame to obtain precise measurements of active motion in 121 healthy adult subjects (Table 13.2). Females had a greater range of plantar flexion, whereas males had a greater range of dorsiflexion. Older males showed a greater decrease in plantar flexion, whereas older females had a greater decrease in the dorsiflexion range. The authors speculated that wearing high-heel shoes and differences in physical activity caused differences in ankle motion.

TABLE 13.2

COMPARISON OF ANKLE MOTION WITH GENDER AND AGE*

Gender	Age	Dorsiflexion (Mean ± s.d.)	Plantar Flexion (Mean ± s.d.)
Males	20–59	26.1° ± 6.5°	40.5° ± 8.1°
	60–79	25.9° ± 4.0°	35.0° ± 5.8°
Females	20–59	24.9° + 6.1°	44.4° + 7.7°
	60–79	19.6° + 4.7°	41.2° + 6.5°

*Adapted from Nigg and associates[86]

The landmarks used in clinical measurements of ankle motion alter the degree of measurement. Bohannon and associates[85] observed a significant difference in ankle motion when the axis of measurement was the heel versus the plantar surface of the foot versus the fifth metatarsal. Elveru and associates[87] also found a relatively low correlation coefficient of intertester reliability when measuring passive ankle dorsiflexion (0.50 for ankle dorsiflexion and 0.72 for ankle plantar flexion). Therefore, to minimize variability in measurements, examiners should strive to use consistent landmarks on the foot and leg when measuring ankle motion. In adults and children old enough to cooperate, measuring active motion is preferred, as that method seems to provide more consistency in range of motion, particularly that of dorsiflexion.

C
H A P T E R 1 4

The Foot

Motion of the foot is typically described in the plane of prona-
tion/supination and inversion/eversion. Inversion (turning the
heel inward) and eversion (turning the heel outward) primarily
reflect motion at the talocalcaneal joint. Using a specially constructed frame, Nigg and associates[86] measured subtalar motion
in adults of different ages. Compared to subjects 20 to 59 years
old, the arc of inversion/eversion was decreased by an average
of 6° in those who were 60 to 79 years of age. No significant
difference, however, was observed in females versus males.

The axis of the talocalcaneal (subtalar) joint is oblique with an
average vertical tilt of 42° and an average medial deviation of
16°.[88] Therefore, motion about this joint also includes inter-
nal/external rotation and dorsiflexion/plantar flexion.[89] Clinical
measurements, however, are limited to inversion and eversion.

The oblique axis of the talocalcaneal joint has also engendered
debate concerning the proper Zero Starting Position for measuring inversion and eversion. *Joint Motion: Method of Measuring
and Recording*[33] recommended aligning the heel with the midline of the tibia, but did not specify the position of the ankle.

Cailliet[90] used the same midline axis but positioned the ankle in dorsiflexion. In this position, Milgrom and associates[91] recorded reduced measurement of inversion/eversion. James and associates[92] described a Zero Starting Position that was determined by the neutral position of the subtalar joint, eg, the foot being positioned somewhat oblique to the midline axis of the tibia. Attempting to position the heel with the subtalar axis in neutral lacks precision, and Elveru and associates[87,93] have demonstrated poorer reliability when subtalar joint measurements were based on a subtalar joint neutral position.

We now recommend that the ankle be positioned in gentle dorsiflexion when measuring inversion and eversion (Fig. 14.1-14.3). Dorsiflexion limits lateral motion at the tibiotalar joint, and therefore, that position should better reflect subtalar joint motion. Standardizing the ankle position should also improve the reliability of measurements, as previous studies have demonstrated a rather diverse range of motion when inversion/eversion was measured with the ankle in an unspecified position (Table 14.1). Further studies that measure inversion/eversion with the ankle in a specified position are needed.

An inclinometer may be a better tool for measuring subtalar motion (Fig. 14.4). Mann[94] advocated this method, but we are unaware of any studies that have analyzed the effectiveness of this technique.

Pronation and supination refer to rotation of the foot about an anterior/posterior axis. As such, supination includes inversion of the heel as well as adduction and plantar flexion of the midfoot (Fig. 14.5). Pronation is the opposite motion and includes eversion of the heel and abduction and dorsiflexion of the midfoot (Fig. 14.6).

The movement of pronation and supination occurs at all joints of the foot from the tibiotalar to the tarsometatarsal region.[95] Therefore, it is difficult to quantify pronation and supination of the foot. Useful information, however, can be obtained when motion of an affected foot is compared with that of the unaffected side.

TABLE 14.1

SUBTALAR MOTION: HEALTHY ADULT MALES, ANKLE POSITION UNSPECIFIED

	Boone and Azen[14] (Mean ± s.d.)	Roaas and Andersson[18] (Mean ± s.d.)
Inversion	37° ± 4.5°	28° ± 6.9°
Eversion	21° ± 5.0°	28° ± 4.8°

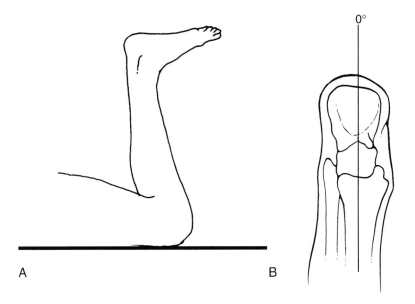

A   B

Fig. 14.1A   **ZERO STARTING POSITION:** The patient is lying prone with the knee flexed, and the ankle in gentle dorsi-flexion, ie, just until the soft tissues become taut.

Fig. 14.1B   Flexion of the knee will place the axis of the subtalar joint close to the horizontal plane.[94]

The Clinical Measurement of Joint Motion

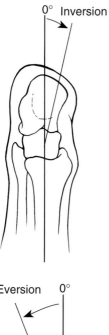

0° Inversion

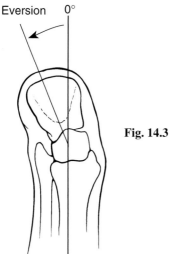

Eversion   0°

Fig. 14.2

INVERSION: The heel is moved medially, and the degree of inversion is measured from the Zero Starting Position.

Fig. 14.3

EVERSION: The heel is moved outward and the degree of motion is measured from the Zero Starting Position.

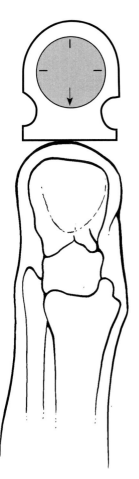

Fig. 14.4 **INCLINOMETER METHOD:** With the heel in the Zero Starting Position, the inclinometer is set at zero. The heel is then moved into maximum inversion and the degree of inclination is recorded. A similar process is repeated for measurement of eversion.

The Clinical Measurement of Joint Motion

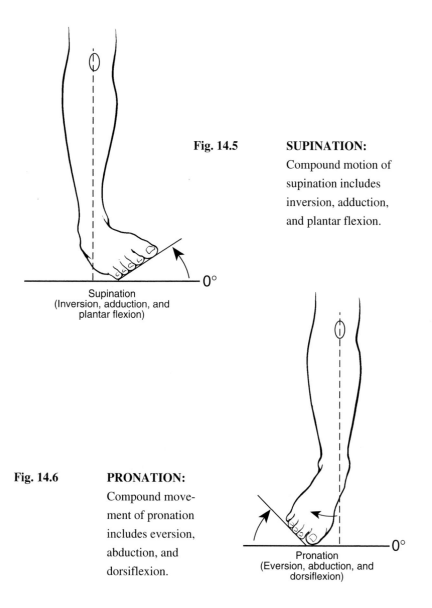

Fig. 14.5

Supination
(Inversion, adduction, and
plantar flexion)

SUPINATION: Compound motion of supination includes inversion, adduction, and plantar flexion.

Fig. 14.6

PRONATION: Compound movement of pronation includes eversion, abduction, and dorsiflexion.

Pronation
(Eversion, abduction, and
dorsiflexion)

CHAPTER 15

The Hallux

The hallux, or great toe, includes the metatarsophalangeal (MTP) joint and the interphalangeal (IP) joint. Motion at both joints is in the dorsiflexion/plantar flexion plane, but dorsiflexion is virtually nonexistent at the IP joint, while plantar flexion is less than dorsiflexion at the MTP joint (Figs. 15.1–15.2).

In *Joint Motion: Method of Measuring and Recording*[33] the Zero Starting Position for measuring MTP motion was the longitudinal axis of the first metatarsal aligned with the longitudinal axis of the proximal phalanx (anatomic neutral position). A subsequent report by a committee from the American Orthopaedic Foot and Ankle Society[96] suggested a Zero Starting Position that aligned the proximal segment of the hallux with the plantar surface of the foot. We agree that this functional neutral position is a better Zero Starting Position for measuring motion at the MTP joint of the hallux. It is easier to measure, facilitates description of toe movement during walking, and is similar to the Zero Starting Position of the ankle.

As compared with the anatomic neutral position, using the functional neutral position will make dorsiflexion at the MTP joint comparatively less and plantar flexion comparatively more. Although we are unaware of studies documenting this comparative difference, it would probably be in the range of 20° to 25°. This assumption is based on the study by Steel and associates[97] that measured standing radiographs of 41 normal adult females and found that the first metatarsal-plantar surface angle averaged 22° ± 1.5°.

We are unaware of clinical studies that have documented the normal range of motion of either the MTP or IP joint of the hallux. Shereff and associates[98] did perform radiographic kinematic analysis on six normal amputation specimens. In this study, the total arc of motion averaged 110° at the MTP joint.

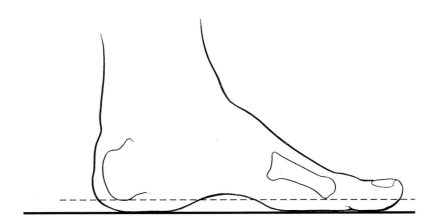

Fig. 15.1   **ZERO STARTING POSITION FOR MEASURING
METATARSOPHALANGEAL MOTION OF
THE HALLUX:** The hallux is placed in the functional
neutral position by aligning the great toe with the plantar
surface of the foot. The plane defining the plantar surface
of the foot is based on an imaginary line connecting the
calcaneal tuberosity and the head of the first metatarsal.

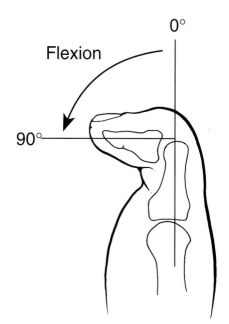

Fig. 15.2   **HALLUX INTERPHALANGEAL JOINT:** The Zero
Starting Position is the longitudinal axis of the distal phalanx
aligned with the longitudinal axis of the proximal phalanx.
Virtually no dorsiflexion occurs at the interphalangeal joint.

The Toes

Movement of the second to fifth toes is similar to motion at the index through little fingers. Flexion occurs at the metatarsal phalangeal (MP), proximal interphalangeal (PIP) and distal interphalangeal (DIP) joints of the toes (Fig. 16.1). Extension occurs at the MP joints. Limited abduction and adduction also take place in the toes (Fig. 16.2).

Although toe motion can be measured and expressed in degrees, this is rarely done in the clinical setting. Not only are measurements of toe motion difficult to perform, but they also have limited usefulness. Visual estimation of flexibility and contractures is usually sufficient at the toes, but defining abnormal postures is also helpful. For example, a **claw toe** is characterized by hyperextension at the MP joint, and flexion contractures of both the PIP and DIP joints. A **hammer toe** has a flexion contracture at the PIP joint, a less severe extension contracture at the MP joint, but no contractures at the DIP joint. A **mallet toe** deformity is limited to a flexion contracture at the DIP joint.

The Clinical Measurement of Joint Motion

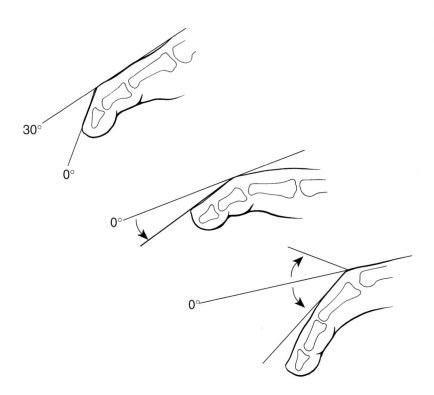

Fig. 16.1 **SECOND TO FIFTH TOES:** Flexion and extension at the toe joints can be measured in a manner similar to measuring finger joint motion.

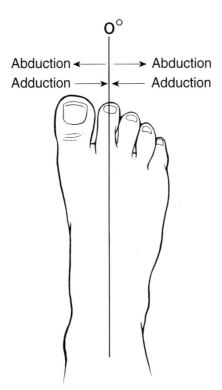

Fig. 16.2   **ABDUCTION AND ADDUCTION:** This is measured in
relationship to the second toe, which is the midline axis of
the foot.

Clinical Measurement of Joint Alignment

Goniometric measurement of joint alignment can be a valuable and practical part of the musculoskeletal examination, especially at the elbow, knee, and hallux. The technique of measuring alignment at these three joints will be described, but the principles of these measurements can also be applied to other joints as well as to angular deformities of the skeleton. Similar to joint motion, joint alignment measurements should be compared with an unaffected side whenever possible.

Varus and valgus are the terms used to define alignment in the coronal plane. Varus means that the distal segment is deviated toward the midline of the body, whereas valgus means that the distal segment is deviated away from the midline. Varus or valgus angulation is expressed in degrees.

Some degree of valgus alignment is normal at the elbow, a posture that is typically described as cubitus valgus or the carrying angle. Clinical measurement of the carrying angle is performed with the elbow in full extension as flexion decreases the degree of cubitus valgus[35](Fig. 17.1).

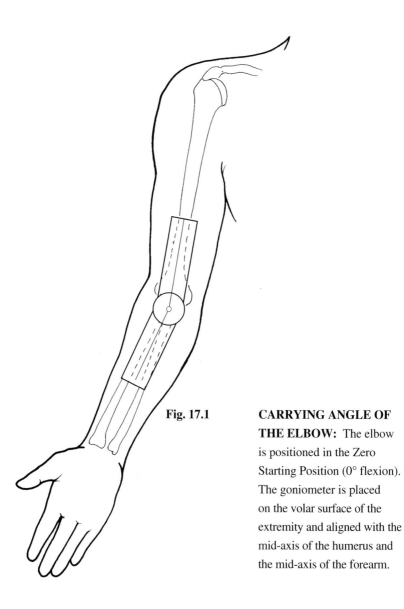

Fig. 17.1

CARRYING ANGLE OF THE ELBOW: The elbow is positioned in the Zero Starting Position (0° flexion). The goniometer is placed on the volar surface of the extremity and aligned with the mid-axis of the humerus and the mid-axis of the forearm.

Baughman and associates[99] made clinical measurements of the carrying angle in 100 adults and found a significant difference between females (14.8° ± 0.7° valgus) and males (10.7° ± 0.8° valgus). On the other hand, two studies[101,102] that measured the carrying angle on radiographs did not find a difference in gender. To explain the difference in clinical and radiographic studies, Beals[100] speculated that hyperextension of the elbow was more frequent in females and that this posture was prevented when radiographs were made.

The technique of measuring knee joint alignment is outlined in Figure 17.2. Goniometric measurements of the anatomic (distal femoral-proximal tibial) axis of the knee are sufficient for most clinical evaluations, but prior to an osteotomy or total joint arthroplasty, radiographs that allow measurement of the mechanical (hip-knee-ankle) axis are preferred.

Knee alignment varies considerably as children develop. It progresses from 10° to 15° of varus at birth to a neutral femoral-tibial alignment at 14 to 22 months of age, to peak valgus angulation of 10° to 15° when the child is 3 to 3.5 years old.[102,103] This maximum valgus then gradually decreases until normal adult alignment is achieved at age 6 to 8 years.

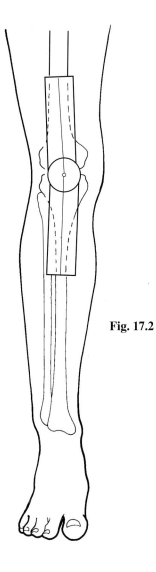

Fig. 17.2

KNEE ALIGNMENT: If possible, knee alignment should be measured with the patient standing and the knee in full extension. The goniometer is aligned with the mid-axis of the distal femur and proximal tibia. In the obese patient, it may be difficult to palpate the distal femur.

Slight valgus is normal at the knee joint in adults. Hsu and associates[104] made detailed measurements on standardized weightbearing radiographs of 120 normal adult subjects and found that the anatomic axis averaged 4.2° ± 1.7° valgus. Gender and age did not affect the degree of genu valgum. Most clinicians, however, have the impression that females have slightly greater valgus alignment of the knee. The relatively greater width of the pelvis may cause genu valgum to be apparently greater in females, but Hsu's study would indicate that bony alignment is not significantly altered by gender.

Mild valgus is also normal at the metatarsophalangeal joint of the hallux, and valgus angulation at this joint can be markedly accentuated by narrow-toed shoes. Clinical measurements are obtained by aligning the goniometer with the longitudinal axis of the first metatarsal and the longitudinal axis of the proximal phalanx (Fig. 17.3). A hallux valgus of greater than 15° to 20° is considered abnormal, but this degree of angulation does not always cause a symptomatic bunion deformity.[92] Hallux valgus averaged 12° ± 2.4° but ranged from 0° to 32° when Steel and associates[97] made radiographic measurements on 41 asymptomatic adult middle-age females.

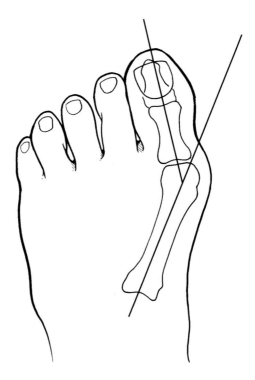

Fig. 17.3   **HALLUX VALGUS:** The goniometer is aligned with the mid-axis of the first metatarsal and the mid-axis of the proximal phalanx. With severe hallux valgus, a concomitant valgus angulation is often noted at the interphalangeal joint of the great toe. This deformity should be recorded as a separate measurement.

References

1. Altman RD: Criteria for the classification of osteoarthritis of the knee and hip. *Scand J Rheumatol Suppl* 1987;65:31-39.

2. Greene WB, Yankaskas BC, Guilford WB: Roentgenographic classifications of hemophilic arthropathy: Comparison of three systems and correlation with clinical parameters. *J Bone Joint Surg* 1989;71A:237-244.

3. Johnson RP, Babbitt DP: Five stages of joint disintegration compared with range of motion in hemophilia. *Clin Orthop* 1985;201:36-42.

4. Kirchheimer JC, Wanivenhaus A: Declines in the range of motion and malalignment in hands of patients with juvenile rheumatoid arthritis studied over 6 years. *J Rheumatol* 1990;17:1653-1656.

5. Parker JW, Harrell PB, Alarcon GS: The value of the joint alignment and motion scale in rheumatoid arthritis. *J Rheumatol* 1988;15:1212-1215.

6. Spiegel TM, Spiegel JS, and Paulus HE: The joint alignment and motion scale: A simple measure of joint deformity in patients with rheumatoid arthritis. *J Rheumatol* 1987;14:887-892.

7. Engelberg AL (ed): *Guides to the Evaluation of Permanent Impairment,* ed 3. Chicago, IL, American Medical Association, 1988.

8. Watkins MA, Riddle DL, Lamb RL, et al: Reliability of goniometric measurements and visual estimates of knee range of motion obtained in a clinical setting. *Phys Ther* 1991;71:90-97.

9. Cave EF, Roberts SM: A method for measuring and recording joint function. *J Bone Joint Surg* 1936;18:455-465.

10. Cheng JC, Chan PS, Hui PW: Joint laxity in children. *J Pediatr Orthop* 1991;11:752-756.

11. Wynne-Davies R: Familial joint laxity. *Proc R Soc Med* 1971; 64:689-690.

12. Ahlberg A, Moussa M, Al-Nahdi M: On geographical variations in the normal range of joint motion. *Clin Orthop* 1988;234:229-231.

13. Boone DC, Azen SP, Lin C-M, et al: Reliability of goniometric measurements. *Phys Ther* 1978;58:1355-1390.

14. Boone DC, Azen SP: Normal range of motion of joints in male subjects. *J Bone Joint Surg* 1979;61A:756-759.

15. Hamilton GF, Lachenbruch PA: Reliability of goniometers in assessing finger joint angle. *Phys Ther* 1969;49:465-469.

16. Murray MP, Gore DR, Gardner GM, et al: Shoulder motion and muscle strength of normal men and women in two age groups. *Clin Orthop* 1985;192:268-273.

17. Mallon WJ, Brown HR, Nunley JA: Digital ranges of motion: Normal values in young adults. *J Hand Surg* 1991;73A:882-887.

18. Roaas A, Andersson GB: Normal range of motion of the hip, knee and ankle joints in male subjects, 30-40 Years of Age. *Acta Orthop Scand* 1982;53:205-208.

19. Svenningsen S, Terjesen T, Auflem M, et al: Hip motion related to age and sex. *Acta Orthop Scand* 1989;60:97-100.

20. Shaw SJ, Morris MA: The range of motion of the metacarpophalangeal joint of the thumb and its relationship to injury. *J Hand Surg* 1992;17B:164-166.

21. Clapper MP, Wolf SL: Comparison of the reliability of the Orthoranger and the standard goniometer for assessing active lower extremity range of motion. *Phys Ther* 1988;68:214-218.

References

22. Dvorak J, Antinnes JA, Panjabi M, et al: Age and gender related normal motion of the cervical spine. *Spine* 1992;17(suppl 10):S393-S398.

23. Battie MC, Bigos SJ, Fisher LD, et al: The role of spinal flexibility in back pain complaints within industry. A prospective study. *Spine* 1990;15:768-773.

24. Roach KE, Miles TP: Normal hip and knee active range of motion: The relationship to age. *Phys Ther* 1991;71:656-665.

25. Baxter MP: Assessment of normal pediatric knee ligament laxity using the genucom. *J Pediatr Orthop* 1988;8:546-550.

26. Forero N, Okamura LA, Larson MA: Normal ranges of hip motion in neonates. *J Pediatr Orthop* 1989;9:391-395.

27. Hoffer MM: Joint motion limitation in newborns. *Clin Orthop* 1980; 148:94-96.

28. Coon V, Donato G, Houser C, et al: Normal ranges of hip motion in infants six weeks, three months and six months of age. *Clin Orthop* 1975;110:256-260.

29. Staheli LT, Corbett M, Wyss C, et al: Lower-extremity rotational problems in children: Normal values to guide management. *J Bone Joint Surg* 1985;67A:39-47.

30. Hoaglund FT, Yau AC, Wong WL: Osteoarthritis of the hip and other joints in southern Chinese in Hong Kong. *J Bone Joint Surg* 1973;55A:545-557.

31. Reid DC, Burnham RS, Saboe LA, et al: Lower extremity flexibility patterns in classical ballet dancers and their correlation to lateral hip and knee injuries. *Am J Sports Med* 1987;15:347-352.

32. Browne AO, Hoffmeyer P, Tanaka S, et al: Glenohumeral elevation studied in three dimensions. *J Bone Joint Surg* 1990;72B:843-845.

33. The Committee for the Study of Joint Motion (eds): *Joint Motion: Method of Measuring and Recording*. Chicago, IL, American Academy of Orthopaedic Surgeons, 1965.

34. Kronberg M, Brostrom L-A, Soderlund V: Retroversion of the humeral head in the normal shoulder and its relationship to the normal range of motion. *Clin Orthop* 1990;253:113-117.

35. An KN, Morrey BF: Biomechanics of the elbow, in Morrey BF (ed): *The Elbow and its Disorders*, Philadelphia, PA, WB Saunders Company, 1985, chap 3, pp 43-61.

36. Petherick M, Rheault W, Kimble S, et al: Concurrent validity and intertester reliability of universal and fluid-based goniometers for active elbow range of motion. *Phys Ther* 1988;68:966-969.

37. Morrey BF, Askew LJ, Chao EY: A biomechanical study of normal functional elbow motion. *J Bone Joint Surg* 1981;63A:872-877.

38. Wagner C: Determination of the rotary flexibility of the elbow joint. *Eur J Appl Physiol* 1977;37:47-59.

39. Sarrafian SK, Melamed JL, Goshgarian GM: Study of wrist motion in flexion and extension. *Clin Orthop* 1977;126:153-159.

40. Ryu JY, Cooney WP III, Askew LJ, et al: Functional ranges of motion of the wrist joint. *J Hand Surg* 1991;16A:409-419.

41. Volz RG, Lieb M, Benjamin J: Biomechanics of the wrist. *Clin Orthop* 1980;149:112-117.

42. Swanson AB, Goran-Hagert C, de-Groot-Swanson G: Evaluation of impairment in the upper extremity. *J Hand Surg* 1987;12A:896-926.

43. Hume MC, Gellman H, McKellop H, et al: Functional range of motion of the joints of the hand. *J Hand Surg* 1990;15A:240-243.

References

44. Johnson RM, Hart DL, Simmons EF, et al: Cervical orthoses: A study comparing their effectiveness in restricting cervical motion in normal subjects. *J Bone Joint Surg* 1977;59A:332-339.

45. Dvorak J, Hayek J, Zehnder R: CT-functional diagnostics of the rotatory instability of the upper cervical spine: Part 2: An evaluation on healthy adults and patients with suspected instability. *Spine* 1987;12:726-731.

46. Penning L, Wilmink JT: Rotation of the cervical spine: A CT study in normal subjects. *Spine* 1987;12: 732-738.

47. Panjabi M, Dvorak J, Duranceau J, et al: Three-dimensional movements of the upper cervical spine. *Spine* 1988;13:726-730.

48. Dvorak J, Panjabi MM, Novotny JE, et al: In vivo flexion/extension of the normal cervical spine. *J Orthop Res* 1991;9:828-834.

49. Mimura M, Moriya H, Watanabe T, et al: Three-dimensional motion analysis of the cervical spine with special reference to the axial rotation. *Spine* 1989;14:1135-1139.

50. Alund M, Larsson SE: Three-dimensional analysis of neck motion: A clinical method. *Spine* 1990;15:87-91.

51. Dvorak J, Panjabi MM, Grob D, et al: Clinical validation of functional flexion/extension radiographs of the cervical spine. *Spine* 1993;18:120-127.

52. Youdas JW, Carey JR, Garrett TR: Reliability of measurements of cervical spine range of motion—comparison of three methods. *Phys Ther* 1991;71:98-106.

53. Einkauf DK, Gohdes ML, Jensen GM, et al: Changes in spinal mobility with increasing age in women. *Phys Ther* 1987;67:370-375.

54. Fitzgerald GK, Wynveen KJ, Rheault W, et al: Objective assessment with establishment of normal values for lumbar spinal range of motion. *Phys Ther* 1983;63:1776-1781.

55.   Loebl WY: Measurement of spinal posture and range of spinal movement. *Ann Phys Med* 1967;9:103-110.

56.   Moll JM, Wright V: Normal range of spinal mobility. An objective clinical study. *Ann Rheum Dis* 1971;30:381-386.

57.   Moll JM, Liyanage SP, Wright V: An objective clinical method to measure spinal extension. *Rheumatol Phys Med* 1972;11:293-312.

58.   Dvorak J, Panjabi MM, Chang DG, et al: Functional radiographic diagnosis of the lumbar spine: Flexion-extension and lateral bending. *Spine* 1991:16:562-571.

59.   Pearcy M, Portek I, Shepherd J: Three-dimensional x-ray analysis of normal movement in the lumbar spine. *Spine* 1984;9:294-297.

60.   Pearcy MJ, Tibrewal SB: Axial rotation and lateral bending in the normal lumbar spine measured by three-dimensional radiography. *Spine* 1984;9:582-587.

61.   Dvorak J, Panjabi MM, Novotny JE, et al: Clinical validation of functional flexion-extension roentgenograms of the lumbar spine. *Spine* 1991;16:943-950.

62.   Gregersen GG, Lucas DB: An in vivo study of the axial rotation of the human thoracolumbar spine. *J Bone Joint Surg* 1967;49A:247-262.

63.   White AA III: Analysis of the mechanics of the thoracic spine in man: An experimental study of autopsy specimens. *Acta Orthop Scand Suppl* 1969;127:1-105.

64.   White AA III, Panjabi MM (eds): Kinematics of the spine, in *Clinical Biomechanics of the Spine*, ed 2. Philadelphia, PA, JB Lippincott Company, 1990.

65.   Williams R, Binkley J, Bloch R, et al: Reliability of the modified-modified Schober and double inclinometer methods for measuring lumbar flexion and extension. *Phys Ther* 1993;73:33-44.

References

66. Gill K, Krag MH, Johnson GB, et al: Repeatability of four clinical methods for assessment of lumbar spinal motion. *Spine* 1988;13:50-53.

67. Schober P: Lendenwirbelsäule und Kreuzschmerzen. *München Med-Wchnschr* 1937;84:336-338.

68. Macrae IF, Wright V: Measurement of back movement. *Ann Rheum Dis* 1969;28:584-589.

69. Hoppenfeld S, Hutton R (eds): *Physical Examination of the Spine and Extremities*, East Norwalk, CT: Appleton-Century-Crofts, 1976.

70. Miller SA, Mayer T, Cox R, et al: Reliability problems associated with the modified Schober technique for true lumbar flexion measurement. *Spine* 1992;17:345-348.

71. van Adrichem JAM, van der Korst JK: Assessment of the flexibility of the lumbar spine. A pilot study in children and adolescents. *Scand J Rheumatol* 1973; 2:87-91.

72. Mayer TG, Tencer AF, Kristoferson S, et al: Use of noninvasive techniques for quantification of spinal range-of-motion in normal subjects and chronic low-back dysfunction patients. *Spine* 1984;9:588-595.

73. Keeley J, Mayer TG, Cox R, et al: Quantification of lumbar function. Part 5: reliability of range-of-motion measures in the sagittal plane and an in vivo torso rotation measurement technique. *Spine* 1986;11:31-35.

74. Portek I, Pearcy MJ, Reader GP, et al: Correlation between radiographic and clinical measurement of lumbar spine movement. *Br J Rheum* 1983;22:197-205.

75. Salisbury PJ, Porter RW: Measurement of lumbar sagittal mobility: A comparison of methods. *Spine* 1987;12:190-193.

76. Beattie P, Rothstein JM, Lamb RL: Reliability of the attraction method for measuring lumbar spine backward bending. *Phys Ther* 1987;67:364-369.

77. Mellin GP: Accuracy of measuring lateral flexion of the spine with a tape. *Clin Biomech* 1986;1:85-89.

78. Boline PD, Keating JC Jr, Haas M, et al: Interexaminer reliability and discriminant validity of inclinometric measurement of lumbar rotation in chronic low-back pain patients and subjects without low-back pain. *Spine* 1992;17:335-338.

79. Haas SS, Epps CH Jr, Adams JP: Normal ranges of hip motion in the newborn. *Clin Orthop* 1973;91:114-118.

80. Waugh KG, Minkel JL, Parker R, et al: Measurement of selected hip, knee, and ankle joint motions in newborns. *Phys Ther* 1983;63:1616-1621.

81. Phelps E, Smith LJ, Hallum A: Normal ranges of hip motion of infants between nine and 24 months of age. *Dev Med Child Neurol* 1985;27:785-792.

82. Lundberg A, Goldie I, Kalin B, et al: Kinematics of the ankle/foot complex: Plantarflexion and dorsiflexion. *Foot Ankle* 1989;9:194-200.

83. Ouzounian TJ, Shereff MJ: In vitro determination of midfoot motion. *Foot Ankle* 1989;10:140-146.

84. Backer M, Kofoed H: Passive ankle mobility: Clinical measurement compared with radiography. *J Bone Joint Surg* 1989;71B:696-698.

85. Bohannon RW, Tiberio D, Zito M: Selected measures of ankle dorsiflexion range of motion: Differences and intercorrelations. *Foot Ankle* 1989;10:99-103.

86. Nigg BM, Fisher V, Allinger TL, et al: Range of motion of the foot as a function of age. *Foot Ankle* 1992;13:336-343.

References

87. Elveru RA, Rothstein JM, Lamb RL: Goniometric reliability in a clinical setting. Subtalar and ankle joint measurements. *Phys Ther* 1988;68:672-677.

88. Manter JT: Movements of the subtalar and transverse tarsal joints. *Anat Rec* 1941;80:397-410.

89. Close JR, Inman VT, Poor PM, et al: The function of the subtalar joint. *Clin Orthop* 1967;50:159-179.

90. Cailliet R (ed): Examination of the foot, in *Foot and Ankle Pain*, ed 2. Philadelphia, PA, FA Davis Company, 1983, chap 2, pp 31-46.

91. Milgrom C, Giladi M, Simkin A, et al: The normal range of subtalar inversion and eversion in young males as measured by three different techniques. *Foot Ankle* 1985;6:143-145.

92. James SL, Bates BT, Osternig LR: Injuries to runners. *Am J Sports Med* 1978;6:40-50.

93. Elveru RA, Rothstein JM, Lamb RL, et al: Methods for taking subtalar joint measurements. A clinical report. *Phys Ther* 1988;68:678-682.

94. Mann, RA: Principles of examination of the foot and ankle, in Mann RA (ed): *Surgery of the Foot: In Memory of Henri L DuVries and Verne T. Inman*, ed 5. St. Louis, MO, CV Mosby Company, 1986, chap 2, pp 31-49.

95. Lundberg A, Svensson OK, Bylund C, et al: Kinematics of the ankle/foot complex: Part 2: Pronation and supination. *Foot Ankle* 1989;9:248-253.

96. Smith RW, Reynolds JC, Stewart MJ: Hallux valgus assessment: Report of research committee of American Orthopaedic Foot and Ankle Society. *Foot Ankle* 1984;5:92-103.

97. Steel MW III, Johnson KA, DeWitz MA, et al: Radiographic measurements of the normal adult foot. *Foot Ankle* 1980;1:151-158.

98.   Shereff MJ, Bejjani FJ, Kummer FJ: Kinematics of the first metatarsopha-langeal joint. *J Bone Joint Surg* 1986;68A:392-398.

99.   Baughman FA Jr, Higgins JV, Wadsworth TG, et al: The carrying angle in sex chromosome anomalies. *JAMA* 1974;230:718-720.

100. Beals RK: The normal carrying angle of the elbow: A radiographic study of 422 patients. *Clin Orthop* 1976;119:194-196.

101. Steel FL, Tomlinson JD: The "carrying angle" in Man. *J Anat* 1958;92:315-317.

102. Engel GM, Staheli LT: The natural history of torsion and other factors influ-encing gait in childhood: A study of the angle of gait, tibial torsion, knee angle, hip rotation, and development of the arch in normal children. *Clin Orthop* 1974;99:12-17.

103. Salenius P, Vankka E: The development of the tibiofemoral angle in children. *J Bone Joint Surg* 1975;57A:259-261.

104. Hsu RW, Himeno S, Coventry MB, et al: Normal axial alignment of the lower extremity and load-bearing distribution at the knee. *Clin Orthop* 1990;255:215-227.